Physical fitness for practically everybody

The Consumers Union Report on Exercise

Physical fitness for practically everybody

The Consumers Union Report on Exercise

by Ivan Kusinitz, Morton Fine,
and the Editors of Consumer Reports Books

Consumers Union, Mount Vernon, New York

Tables 1–2 and 1–9. Adapted from: Brian J. Sharkey, *Fitness and Work Capacity*. United States Department of Argiculture, Forest Service, 1977.

Tables 1–4 and 1–5. Adapted from: Henry J. Montoye, et al., "Heart rate response to a modified Harvard step test: males and females, ages 10-69," *Research Quarterly*, vol. 40, no. 1.

Tables 1–6, A–1, and A–2. Adapted from: Albert M. Kattus, M.D., et al., *Exercise Testing and Training of Apparently Healthy Individuals: A Handbook for Physicians*. American Heart Association, Committee on Exercise, 1972.

Tables 1–7 and 1–8 (and C–1 and C–2). Adapted from: Frank I. Katch and William D. McArdle, *Nutrition, Weight Control and Exercise*. Houghton Mifflin Company, 1977.

Table 1–10. Adapted from: Charles Corbin, et al., *Concepts in Physical Education*. Wm. C. Brown Company, 1978.

Tables 1–11, 1–12, and 5–1. Adapted from: Perry Johnson, et al., *Sports, Exercise and You*. Holt, Rinehart & Winston, 1975.

Tables 1–13 and 1–14. Adapted from: M.L. Pollock, et al., *Health and Fitness through Physical Activity*. John Wiley & Sons, 1978.

Tables 1–15 and 1–16. Adapted from: C.R. Myers, *The Official YMCA Physical Fitness Handbook*. Popular Library, 1977.

Table 3–2. Adapted from: *Beyond Diet...Exercise Your Way to Fitness and Heart Health*. CPC International Inc., 1974.

Appendix B. Adapted from: *Build and Blood Pressure Study, 1959,* Society of Actuaries. Prepared by the Metropolitan Life Insurance Company.

Contents

Tables

Tables

Introduction

With this notice in the August 1978 *Consumer Reports,* we asked readers of the magazine to participate in the preparation of this book.

Wanted: Readers Who Exercise—and Readers Who Don't

Consumers Union invites those who exercise, as well as those who don't, to tell us your views and experiences. Your letters will help us with a book on physical fitness for practically everybody.

■ **If you currently exercise,** please include information on: the type(s) of activity; how often you do each activity; length of each session; how you got started; how long you've been doing the activity; your expectations or goals (and whether any have been accomplished); benefits; injuries incurred; and experiences that might be helpful to others.

■ **If you stopped exercising,** why did you stop? Are you considering resuming? Also, please tell us about your past exercise experience (as above).

■ **If you never tried exercising,** what has kept you from starting?

Please include in your letter any specific concerns you may have about exercise and fitness, your age, sex, state of health, and other information you think relevant. Address your comments to: Consumers Union, Dept. Ex, 256 Washington Street, Mount Vernon, N.Y. 10550.

More than a thousand readers responded. We read every one of their letters—and we quote from a number of them in this book. Letters came

11

from all kinds of exercisers and from a few nonexercisers too. Almost all who wrote to us described their exercise experience, giving us details about the regimen they were following and the results they were getting.

It seemed to us that the vast majority of our correspondents were on the right track with their exercise programs. But we did find some misconceptions about exercise, quite a few concerns about health and physical fitness, and any number of specific questions.

In this book we respond to some of the worries and reservations about exercise expressed in the letters. By setting forth clearly what exercise can and cannot do, we also hope to dispel the misconceptions evident among some who wrote to us. Our primary purposes, however, are to help prospective exercisers start on a sensible program, and to help more experienced exercisers who have had difficulty selecting an appropriate fitness activity or keeping at their exercise program.

The word *exercise* to some people connotes formal, structured, planned physical activities undertaken for the sake of competition, physical therapy, or self-improvement. For others, exercise means a prescribed, fixed series of calisthenics, weight lifting, or laps around the track. To some it's a tennis match or an evening at a bowling alley. But exercise is all of these things—and much more. It begins with the fetus and goes on, in one way or another, throughout life.

The title we selected for this book—*Physical Fitness for Practically Everybody*—embodies our conception of exercise: Almost everybody can benefit from exercise, and most people can enjoy it too. Not only the skilled athlete, the perfectly fit, and the exuberant young are potential exercisers. Just about everyone—active or not—is eligible to give it a try. And there are exercise programs geared to achieve every conceivable fitness goal. The key to success is to choose a program that is likely to suit you, your way of life, and your present level of fitness.

If you follow the suggestions and guidelines in this book, you can succeed with exercise. Two cautions sound throughout: Avoid discomfort by beginning a program appropriate for your current state of health and fitness. And don't overdo—progress slowly for best results. The benefits of exercise can be achieved with moderation, over a period of time. Beginning a fitness program should not entail a major disruption of your life or that of your household. But to get results you need to keep on exercising. If an exercise begins to bore you, consult the book to find a substitute activity. Adapt your program to your health, your interests, and your moods.

How to use this book

Physical Fitness for Practically Everybody can be used in two ways. It can be read straight through, of course, but you can also refer to the contents page and to the index to find sections on activities that particularly interest you and answers to some of your questions.

In Part I, we discuss physical fitness in terms of the five basic components of fitness and present the two basic training principles underlying exercise programs. We help you draw up a personal fitness profile, decide whether medical clearance is necessary, and review the fitness goals you can achieve with exercise. We explain how to use calories as a measure of intensity of exercise.

Part II presents specific exercise options—eight basic model programs to help you get started on exercises that will achieve your fitness goals. We also give you information about some eighty sports and activities. You'll find out the calories you can expect to burn by exercising, how best to chart your progress, and how to keep going should your interest flag.

Part III concentrates on answering some of the many questions we received from readers of *Consumer Reports* about training techniques, health-related matters, and about exercise and children, women, and older people. We also give you some help in selecting a commercial or institutional fitness facility.

In the Glossary of Exercises, you will find the exercises that can help you design a fitness program geared to your specific goals. There are a variety of exercises with and without equipment. All the exercises are illustrated. There are instructions on how to perform them and a list of the body parts benefited by each exercise.

Kusinitz and Fine

Ivan Kusinitz, Ph.D., is former chairman of and professor in the Department of Health and Physical Education at York College of the City University of New York. During the Korean War, Kusinitz was officer-in-charge of physical reconditioning at a large United States Air Force hospital. He maintains a lifelong interest in hiking, backpacking, and skiing and currently serves as Education Chairman of the Adirondack Mountain Club. He has climbed all forty-eight peaks over 4,000 feet in New York State and is a member of the Adirondack 46ers.

Morton Fine, Ed.D., is former coordinator of health education and associate professor in the Department of Health and Physical Education at York College of the City University of New York. For many years, he has worked on behalf of young people's running programs and has coached at the high school and college level. He keeps in shape by jogging, swimming, weight training, and cross-country skiing.

Kusinitz and Fine have developed, taught, and supervised fitness programs for children and adults in schools, colleges, and camps. For more than fifteen years, they have collaborated on health education and fitness projects and publications, including such diverse areas as the development of physical fitness, sex education, and cardiac rehabilitation. They also consult on health promotion programs for people with special health and fitness needs, including diabetics, prenatal and post-

13

partum women, cardiac patients, asthmatics, the overweight, and those with sports injuries.

Kusinitz and Fine are grateful to their colleagues in the Department of Health and Physical Education at York College of the City University of New York for their help and support, and to the students of York College from whom they learned much over the years.

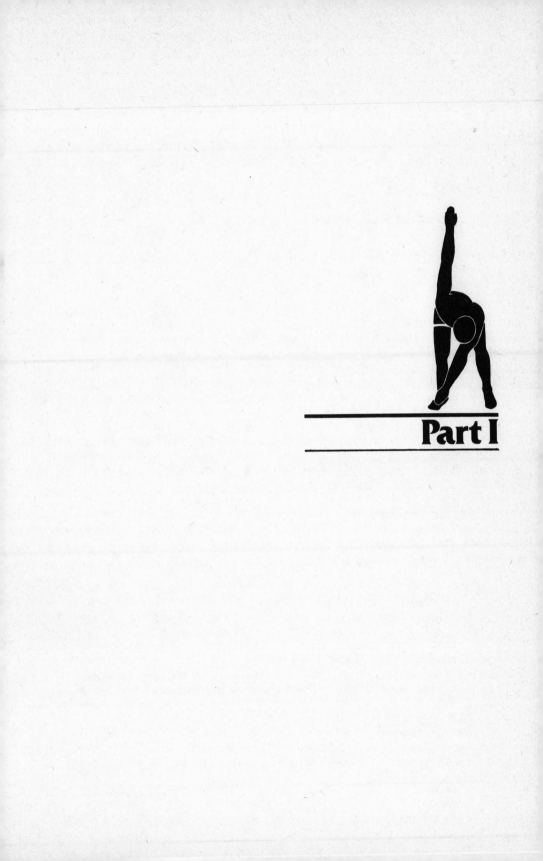

Part I

1

How Fit Are You?

If you're unsure about physical fitness—what it is, how to achieve it, how fit you need to be, and how it relates to good health—you're not the only one. Consider, for example, P.N., a *Consumer Reports* reader from Staten Island, New York, who researched the matter some years ago and thought out his own goals and requirements. Every weekday he runs five or six miles in about forty minutes, preceded and followed by about three minutes of stretching exercises; twice a week he also does a series of weight lifting exercises. But even P.N.—who at age thirty-one stands 6 feet, weighs 170 pounds, has a resting pulse of 50, hasn't been ill for years and, above all, feels good—does not think he's qualified to answer the seemingly simple question, "What is physical fitness?".

To some, physical fitness is a sacred article of faith, an eternal verity. John F. Kennedy ranked it along with mental, moral, and spiritual fitness as essential to the nation's strength. According to one college textbook, physical fitness contributes to the "unitary...holistic nature" of the human organism. At the opposite end of the spectrum are the people who think physical fitness is something for others to work at (combat soldiers, say, or professional athletes and their coaches). Some sedentary types may share the discomfort of S.R. of Princeton, New Jersey, who told Consumers Union, "I see joggers by the sweat-sock-full agonizing past my window, and I feel guilty, possibly un-American, about my sluggish life-style." Others eschew guilt and agree with Robert M. Hutchins, former University of Chicago president, who is supposed to have said that whenever he felt the desire to exercise, he lay down until the feeling passed.

Between the extremes, of course, are the great majority who agree that, however hard it may be to define, physical fitness is a desirable condition to be cultivated in a variety of ways and for a variety of reasons. In that large group belong most of the people who reported on exercise to Consumers Union. They include the following exercisers.

■ In hopes of growing old gracefully and comfortably, S.M., a retired

16

seventy-three-year-old Californian said he does calisthenics at home.

■ Having recovered from a heart attack, S.R. of Port Jervis, New York, regularly walks or rides a bicycle to improve his cardiorespiratory endurance.

■ Lifting weights and playing badminton helps thirty-one-year-old A.D. of Pontiac, Michigan, feel and look better (he also believes the exercises may help him live longer).

■ A husband who likes slim women is the incentive thirty-five-year-old D.S. of Coleman, Alabama, needed to stick to running every day to keep in shape.

■ Seventy-five-year-old L.M. of Glencoe, Illinois, swings from her garage roof to reduce the pain and discomfort caused by arthritis.

■ S.N., a "confirmed runner" from Croton, New York, competes against his own goals: "I win only against myself and for myself." At age forty-one, he has "growing old with quality" on his mind.

■ A wife who made remarks about his potbelly induced J.P., a schoolteacher in Portage, Indiana, to start exercising at age forty-nine.

What physical fitness is *not,* clearly, is the same thing for everyone—a precise, readily definable entity with a single fixed standard to be applied universally.

One useful approach to understanding physical fitness has been suggested by the President's Council on Physical Fitness and Sports. Based on the Council's approach, physical fitness can be characterized as the ability to carry out daily tasks without becoming fatigued and with ample energy left to enjoy regular leisure-time pursuits and to handle an occasional unexpected emergency requiring physical exertion. The Council's definition also encompasses the ability to last, to bear up, and to persevere under difficult circumstances.

The Council describes a scale of physical fitness, ranging from "abundant life" at one extreme to "death" at the other. If you're alive, according to this view, you have at least some degree of physical fitness. Admittedly, that degree could be minimal for the severely ill or handicapped. In the highly trained athlete, of course, the degree of physical fitness would be maximal. And it could even vary in the same person at different times. Your own level of fitness is probably shaped to a great extent by your routine—the needs of your job, your sports interests, the stairs you climb, or your twice-daily run for the train.

The physical fitness continuum

The full spectrum of physical fitness can be envisioned as a continuum—a horizontal line on which each individual's physical fitness level is slotted in the appropriate point (see Table 1–1). At the extreme left are those who need help to perform the routine chores of daily life. At the extreme right are healthy athletes, trained and conditioned for competi-

Table 1–1

Physical Fitness Continuum

Low level of fitness					High level of fitness
1	2	3	4	5	6
Need help to function.	Just able to get around; unfit for work or active leisure.	Tired at end of day; no energy left for active leisure.	Minimum energy left at end of day for active leisure.	Energy left at end of day for wide variety of vigorous activities.	Trained athletes.

tion. Others are at the points along the line that reflect their life-style and job requirements.

If you're fit enough to perform the physical activities called for by your way of life, you might be quite content with your place on the fitness continuum. A problem could arise, however, should you take on new activities, need to get back in shape after illness, or misjudge your level of fitness. For those in good condition, a task such as shoveling snow or splitting logs can be invigorating and enjoyable. For those in poor shape, however, a vacation spent skiing may seem like a sentence to hard labor.

Take, for example, two friends who tried cross-country skiing for the first time. One was exhilarated. After a few falls, she got the hang of it and was able to negotiate an easy trail and even attempt a moderate hill. Her friend, on the other hand, was exhausted. For him, the venture was a disaster. It began with his ski pants, last used several years before. They were so tight he had difficulty bending over to fasten his boots to his skis. Climbing a moderate hill and holding his position were difficult. His muscles seemed to "give out," and he fell repeatedly. His arms and legs ached from the unaccustomed motions of striding and reaching. He stopped repeatedly to catch his breath. After fifteen minutes, he felt his limbs grow weary with the weight of clothing and equipment; he was tempted to quit. By the end of the first half hour, he had become so frustrated that he took off his skis and returned to the lodge. Although, like his friend, he had wanted to get outdoors to enjoy the winter landscape, he ended up feeling that cross-country skiing was too much for him.

The more successful of the two cross-country skiers, with her ability to undertake a new and strenuous sport, demonstrated better-than-average fitness. Despite her office job, she would place near 5 on the fitness continuum. Her companion would be more likely to place between 3 and 4. Both, in fact, have sedentary jobs, but the woman bikes eleven miles to and from work every day and plays tennis twice a week. The man drives to work and jogs a half-mile on Sundays (if the weather is nice). With some changes in his routine, however, he could probably improve his level of fitness enough to enjoy cross-country skiing.

Even severely disabled people can improve their place on the fitness continuum with gradual increases in activity. Consider A.A., a sixty-six-year-old *Consumer Reports* reader from Batavia, New York. Five years earlier he had suffered a stroke that left one leg useless and one arm impaired. Under his physician's supervision, he began a program of rehabilitation almost immediately. To control his hypertension (high blood pressure), he was placed on medication and prescribed a diet. To restore the function of his arm and leg, he began an exercise regimen.

"I started by using a walker," A.A. explained, "and quickly advanced to a cane. My next step was to walk without a cane and then develop faster walking." Before long, he had reached his goal of walking three miles a day—"fast, serious walking," in all kinds of weather. He also bikes ten miles a day, weather permitting, all year round. He reports that he has taught himself to walk with "a very unnoticeable limp" and that the arm and hand have returned to normal—along with his life. He works full time, traveling "all over the world" on vacations with his wife. Despite below-zero winters and deep snow, he keeps up his daily walks, takes care of his house and grounds, and does the painting and decorating himself. In short, wrote A.A., five years after suffering a seriously disabling stroke, "I enjoy every minute of my working day."

Like many people, you may find yourself lower on the fitness continuum than you'd like to be. You may even decide that you're unable to perform on a par with recovered stroke victim A.A. Perhaps your level of physical activity has declined a great deal since you left school, or began to work long hours, or had a baby, or retired from your job. If so, you could be unprepared for vacation pursuits you're tempted to try—or even unable to deal comfortably with the physical demands of your daily life. If you want to improve your physical fitness by increasing your level of activity, the first step to take is to decide whether you need clearance from your physician.

Medical clearance

Before you buy a pair of running shoes or sign up for tennis lessons, you would be wise to consider whether you first need medical clearance. Although almost anyone can benefit from exercise, for some people it could be dangerous to suddenly undertake a strenuous program, particularly when the fitness training is unsupervised. For stroke victim A.A., of course, there was no question of proceeding without the approval of his physician. For younger, relatively healthy people who plan to begin a slow and gradual program to improve their physical fitness, would it be necessary to get a physician's advice? Is medical clearance necessary for everyone?

Consumers Union's medical consultants suggest that you can decide this for yourself. First, answer the questions below; then apply the guidelines that follow. After that, you will be ready to assess your level of fitness.

Questions on medical history

A. Read carefully all of questions 1 through 6.
    1. Have you ever had:
        a. A heart attack?
        b. Rapid, irregular heart action or palpitations?
        c. Pain, pressure, or a tight feeling in the chest during exercise or any other physical activity, including sex?
    2. Have you ever taken:
        a. Digitalis?
        b. Nitroglycerin?
        c. Quinidine?
        d. Any other medication for your heart?
    3. Have you ever been told by a physician that you have:
        a. Angina pectoris?
        b. Fibrillation or tachycardia?
        c. An abnormal electrocardiogram (EKG)?
        d. Heart murmur?
        e. Rheumatic heart disease?
        f. Any other heart trouble?
    4. Do you have any of the following risk factors for coronary heart disease?
        a. Do you have diabetes?
        b. Do you have hypertension?
        c. Has your physician ever put you on a special diet for your heart or blood pressure, or given you medication to lower your blood cholesterol level?
        d. Do you have a blood relative who had a heart attack before age sixty?
        e. Do you smoke cigarettes?
    5. Are you more than 20 pounds overweight?
    6. Do you have other health problems that might affect a fitness program?
        a. Do you have any chronic illness?
        b. Do you have asthma, emphysema, or any other lung condition?
        c. Do you get short of breath with activities that don't seem to bother other people?
        d. Have you ever gotten cramps in your legs if you walk briskly?

    e. Do you have arthritis, rheumatism, or gouty arthritis?

    f. Do you have any condition limiting the motion of your muscles, joints, or any part of the body, which could be aggravated by exercise?

B. If you answered "yes" to *any* of questions 1 through 6 you should consult your physician before beginning a fitness program. If you answered "no" to *all* the questions covering your medical history, proceed to the guidelines below.

Guidelines for medical clearance

A. In general, if you are under thirty-five, have no physical complaints, and have had a medical checkup within the past two years, it is probably safe for you—without any special clearance from your physician —to begin exercising at your current level of physical activity and gradually increase it.

B. Regardless of your age, if you are not feeling altogether well, or if you have any specific health concerns, you should get a medical evaluation and clearance from your physician before making any major change in your current level of physical activity.

C. After the age of thirty-five, medical clearance is advisable under certain conditions before you begin a fitness program.

    ■ If you have a history of coronary heart disease, or any of the risk factors for coronary heart disease (see page 20), your physician may require you to undergo a cardiac stress test (exercise tolerance test) before beginning a fitness program.

    ■ If you are unsure whether you have any of the risk factors, you should touch base with your physician and inquire about the advisability of a checkup.

    ■ Although obesity is not a primary risk factor for coronary disease, Consumers Union's medical consultants believe that an individual more than twenty pounds overweight requires clearance before undertaking a fitness and weight control regimen.

    ■ If you have no coronary risk factors, the question of whether you need medical clearance may depend on the nature and extent of the changes you are considering in your daily routine. If you have been exercising regularly, you should be able to increase your level of activity *gradually* without incurring any health problems. (Using the activity index below and the formula on page 23 can help you decide this, should you have any questions.) However, if you have not been exercising on a regular basis, you may wish to take the conservative route and consult your physician. For some sedentary people, such consultation would be mandatory even before beginning to assess physical fitness (see pages 26–41). For someone whose main reason for walking is to head toward the dinner table, such fitness testing may constitute too great an increase in daily activity.

Estimating your level of activity

If you answered "no" to all the questions covering your medical history and if you are already somewhat active, it is probably safe for you to begin a gradual exercise program without medical clearance. The first step would be to assess your physical fitness using the tests described at the end of this chapter. Like many people, you may not be sure how to judge whether you are "somewhat" active.

How does your daily stroll with the dog or your weekly tennis game rate? To make a simple estimate of how active you are, examine your current exercise patterns. Use Table 1–2 to score your current exercise patterns in terms of intensity (how hard), duration (how long), and frequency (how often). Then multiply these scores to get an estimate of your level of activity.

Table 1–2

Activity Index

Your activity index is based on the intensity, duration, and frequency of your current exercise patterns. Rate how hard, how long, and how often you exercise according to the criteria listed below. Then calculate your activity index, using the formula at the end of the table (intensity × duration × frequency = activity index). Suppose you are a skilled tennis player. Your intensity score for competitive singles would be 4; if the match lasts for an hour or more each time, your duration score would be 5; if you play regularly twice a week, your frequency score would be 2. Multiply $4 \times 5 \times 2$ to get your activity index of 40 (moderate active). If, however, your exercise is limited to playing golf twice a week in a foursome that walks through the course, and you carry your own clubs, your index would be 20 $(2 \times 5 \times 2)$, or low active.

How Hard Do You Exercise?

If your exercise results in:	Your intensity score is:
No change in pulse from resting level	0
Little change in pulse from resting level —as in slow walking, bowling, yoga	1
Slight increase in pulse and breathing —as in table tennis, active golf (no golf cart)	2
Moderate increase in pulse and breathing —as in leisurely bicycling, easy continuous swimming, rapid walking	3

22

| Intermittent heavy breathing and sweating
—as in tennis singles, basketball, squash | 4 |
| Sustained heavy breathing and sweating
—as in jogging, cross-country skiing, rope skipping | 5 |

How Long Do You Exercise?

If each session continues for:	Your duration score is:
Less than 5 minutes	0
5 to 14 minutes	1
15 to 29 minutes	2
30 to 44 minutes	3
45 to 59 minutes	4
60 minutes or more	5

How Often Do You Exercise?

If you exercise:	Your frequency score is:
Less than 1 time a week	0
1 time a week	1
2 times a week	2
3 times a week	3
4 times a week	4
5 or more times a week	5

Intensity × Duration × Frequency = Activity Index

Assessing your activity index. Here's how you can translate your activity index into your estimated level of activity.

If your activity index is:	Your estimated level of activity is:
Less than 15	Sedentary
15–24	Low active
25–40	Moderate active
41–60	Active
Over 60	High active

23

Your activity index provides a rough estimate of your current level of activity and a very rough indication of your physical fitness. Its main purpose, at this point, is to help you decide whether it is safe to proceed to a more strenuous—and far more accurate—assessment of your physical fitness.

If your index is 15 or more, it's probably safe to take on the self-assessment tests. But, if you score less than 15 (sedentary), you would be well advised to consult your physician before proceeding to do the self-assessment tests.

The activity index can also help you decide whether you can safely increase your usual round of physical activities. If your current schedule of activities gives you an index of 41 or more (active to high active), you are probably sufficiently fit to enjoy a wide variety of vigorous activities. Increasing your exercise program would probably cause little strain. If your index is between 25 and 40 (moderate active), then you should proceed a little more slowly. If, however, your index is between 15 and 24 (low active), approach any significant increase in activity very gradually and with caution.

Indeed, if before their vacation the two novice cross-country skiers had used the activity index for even a rough assessment of their state of physical fitness, the one who experienced frustration and failure might have realized he would be too out of shape to enjoy so strenuous an outing. And if he had also taken the battery of self-assessment tests described later in this chapter, he would have found out that it was inadequacies in the five major components of physical fitness that led to his failure as a cross-country skier.*

The five components of fitness

Although differences of opinion persist as to how best to define physical fitness, most authorities have come to agree that physical fitness can best be measured by performance in five components: cardiorespiratory endurance, body composition, muscular strength, muscular endurance, and flexibility (see Table 1–3).

The experiences of the cross-country skiers demonstrate how people can differ in terms of the components of physical fitness. The out-of-shape skier had difficulties with all five of them. His shortness of breath indicates lack of *cardiorespiratory endurance* (CRE)—the ability to perform moderately strenuous activity over an extended period of time. CRE is a measure of how well the heart and lungs supply the body's increased need for oxygen during sustained physical effort.

---

*Factors that are not health-related that affect successful participation in a sport such as cross-country skiing include balance, agility, coordination, and speed—all having to do with motor ability, not physical fitness.

Table 1–3

The Five Components of Physical Fitness

Physical fitness component	Definition
Cardiorespiratory endurance	Ability to do moderately strenuous activity over an extended period of time at less than maximum effort.
Body composition	Percentage of the body that is fat.
Muscular strength	Ability to exert maximum force in a single exertion.
Muscular endurance	Ability to repeat movements over and over or to hold a particular position for a prolonged period.
Flexibility	Ability to move a joint easily through its full range of motion.

Sensations of heaviness and clumsiness and the feeling that clothes no longer fit properly reflect *body composition*—the relative proportion of fat to bone and muscle. A professional athlete probably has a more favorable body composition (less fat and more muscle) than a retired office worker, even though their height and weight may be the same.

The skier's failure to climb a moderate hill with ease and to hold his position shows lack of *muscular strength*—the ability to exert maximun force, usually in a single exertion. Lifting a heavy weight or taking a step up the side of a mountain is a measure of muscular strength.

A feeling of exhaustion and the sensation that muscles seem to "give out" relate to lack of *muscular endurance*: the ability to repeat a particular action many times, or hold a particular position for an extended time. With greater endurance, it is less likely your body will feel sore or muscle-bound after exercising. If you have the muscular strength to do one sit-up yet cannot do five, it is probably muscular endurance that is the limiting factor.

Restrictions in movement are likely when there is limited *flexibility*, which is the ability to flex and extend each joint, such as the elbow or the knee, through its maximum range of motion. To proceed up even a moderate hill, a skier needs some flexibility in the hips, knees, and ankles. To manipulate a ski pole, a skier needs flexibility in the shoulders, elbows, and wrists.

The successful cross-country skier, with her ability to undertake a new and strenuous sport, demonstrates better-than-average CRE. Her body composition is relatively lean and muscular, not fat and flabby. Despite spending most of her day at an office job, her muscular strength and endurance are adequate and her joints are flexible. In short, she's in pretty good condition and would rate well on all five of the fitness components.

Assessing your physical fitness

If you've conscientiously answered the questions on medical history, and applied the guidelines on page 21, and then estimated your activity index, you know whether you should try self-testing. If it's medically safe for you to proceed, you will be able to make a relatively simple self-assessment of your physical fitness by taking a series of tests evaluating the five major components of physical fitness. On Table 1–17 (see pages 40–41) you will find space to note the results of these tests as well as any comments you'd like to record.

Cardiorespiratory endurance

The primary component of physical fitness, CRE is a measure of the ability of the heart and lungs to support moderately strenuous activity over an extended period of time.* At all levels of activity, from sleep to running, it is the cardiorespiratory system that transports oxygen from inhaled air through the bloodstream to the working muscles of the body.

Your pulse before getting out of bed in the morning might be 60 beats per minute or lower. As the day progresses with its usual round of activities, your pulse tends to fluctuate as activity levels change. The more strenuous the activity, the more oxygen is needed and the harder the cardiorespiratory system must work. In a person with high CRE, the muscles used in a CRE activity will be more effective at extracting oxygen from the blood than in a person with low CRE. And when CRE is high, the heart and lungs work less hard for any given activity level than when CRE is low (see page 27).

If occasional vigorous activity or some relatively light daily task leaves you panting with your heart pounding for more that just a few minutes, you probably have inadequate CRE. Low CRE is most often associated with inactivty, aging, obesity, illness, and smoking.

The most accurate way to evaluate CRE is to measure the amount of oxygen actually used during strenuous exercise. This measurement can be done at the same time as a cardiac stress test, making use of a treadmill or a stationary bicycle ergometer (an apparatus used in stress testing). During the exercise your breath may be directly analyzed, or, more commonly, oxygen consumption is computed from work load and heart rate measurement.

---

*The terms aerobic endurance and aerobic fitness are sometimes used synonymously with CRE.

The cardiac stress test makes use of elaborate equipment, requires professional supervision and evaluation, and is costly. For many people about to begin an exercise program, such precise measurement of CRE is not necessary. By taking your pulse before and after strenuous exercise, you can make your own rough evaluation of your CRE because there is a close correlation between CRE and the heart rate response to exercise. For most people, the faster the pulse for a given intensity and duration of exercise, the less efficient the cardiorespiratory system is in delivering oxygen to the body. The slower the pulse for that amount of exercise, the higher your CRE. When CRE is high, you not only perform more efficiently but your pulse returns to a resting level more quickly after exercise.

Taking the modified step test will give you a test of CRE that you can use to begin your self-evaluation. But take the test only if you have none of the health problems listed on pages 20–21, and if your activity index—see Table 1–2—is at least 15 (low active). The original Harvard Step Test, developed at the Harvard Fatigue Laboratory, has been modified somewhat in the description below. Designed for ages ten to sixty-nine, the modified step test is based on the fact that the heart rate of someone who is physically fit increases less during exercise and returns to normal faster after exercise than does the heart rate of someone who is not physically fit. To take the modified step test, follow the directions in Table 1–4 and then check your ratings in Table 1–5.

Table 1–4

Modified Step Test

Directions

---

1. Ask someone with a stopwatch or sweep-second hand to time you.

2. At the signal to begin, step up (start with either foot) on a stair or bench that is 8 inches from ground level, and then step down again. Continue stepping up and down, alternating feet, for three consecutive minutes at a rate of 24 steps per minute—about 2 steps every five seconds.

3. Stop at exactly three minutes, and immediately sit in a chair. The active part of the test is now completed.

4. At exactly one minute after you completed the test, count your pulse for thirty seconds (see page 64 for pulse-counting instruction) and multiply by 2 to obtain your one-minute pulse recovery score.

5. Refer to Table 1–5 to determine the rating for your score. If you are unable to step for the full three minutes, consider yourself poor in CRE.

Table 1-5

Ratings for Modified Step Test

The scores below are for heart beats per minute, measured one minute after completion of the modified step test. Ratings for scores are based on age and sex.

Age	Very high	High	Moderate	Low	Very low
Female					
10–19	Below 82	82–90	92–96	98–102	Above 102
20–29	Below 82	82–86	88–92	94–98	Above 98
30–39	Below 82	82–88	90–94	96–98	Above 98
40–49	Below 82	82–86	88–96	98–102	Above 102
50–59	Below 86	86–92	94–98	100–104	Above 104
60–69	Below 86	86–92	94–98	100–104	Above 104
Male					
10–19	Below 72	72–76	78–82	84–88	Above 88
20–29	Below 72	72–78	80–84	86–92	Above 92
30–39	Below 76	76–80	82–86	88–92	Above 92
40–49	Below 78	78–82	84–88	90–94	Above 94
50–59	Below 80	80–84	86–90	92–96	Above 96
60–69	Below 80	80–84	86–90	92–96	Above 96

Assessing your modified step test score. If you are sedentary, your score will probably be around 100 or above, no matter what your age. Conversely, if you're exceptionally fit, your score will be below that of someone your age who is less fit. If your score on the modified step test is well below 100—falling within the very high or high rating—you have high CRE. Chances are you regularly do some activity that enhances CRE. Keep it up. A moderate or low rating indicates there is room for improvement in CRE. If your score falls within the very low rating, then a regular CRE program could make a big difference. Chapter 3 can help you plan a program to increase your CRE, should you so choose. To determine how you're progressing on a CRE program, you may want to use the modified step test on a regular basis. If so, remember to test yourself in the same way and under the same conditions (in the same general health, at the same time of day, at the same interval before or after a meal or vigorous activity, etc.).

Cardiac stress test

If you have had occasion to take a cardiac stress test within the past two to three years, you would have a good way to judge your CRE. Ask your physician or the laboratory that did the test for your oxygen consumption score. See Table 1–6 for an interpretation of your score. (The

---

Table 1–6

Ratings for Oxygen Consumption in Cardiac Stress Test

The scores below are for maximal oxygen consumption (milliliters of oxygen per kilogram of body weight per minute) during a cardiac stress test. Ratings for scores are based on age and sex.

Age	Very high	High	Moderate	Low	Very low
Female					
20–29	Above 48	38–48	31–37	24–30	Below 24
30–39	Above 44	34–44	28–33	20–27	Below 20
40–49	Above 41	31–41	24–30	17–23	Below 17
50–59	Above 37	28–37	21–27	15–20	Below 15
60–69	Above 34	24–34	18–23	13–17	Below 13
Male					
20–29	Above 52	43–52	34–42	25–33	Below 25
30–39	Above 48	39–48	31–38	23–30	Below 23
40–49	Above 44	36–44	27–35	20–26	Below 20
50–59	Above 42	34–42	25–33	18–24	Below 18
60–69	Above 40	31–40	23–30	16–22	Below 16

Assessing your oxygen consumption score. The higher your maximal oxygen consumption, the better your level of CRE. Thus, a score of 48 indicates a higher CRE than a score of 24. If you are generally sedentary, however, your score is likely to be on the low side no matter what your age. (Of course, you can always improve your CRE rating by means of a regular CRE program.) The standards for women are slightly lower than those for men, although an active woman will generally have a higher maximal oxygen consumption than a less active man of the same age.

oxygen consumption score is usually reported in milliliters of oxygen consumed per kilogram of body weight per minute.) If the actual oxygen consumption was not calculated at the time you took the stress test, you can still estimate your score from the data collected during the stress test. Refer to Appendix A, Tables 1 and 2, for the procedure used.

Body composition

The second of the five fitness components, body composition, should not be confused with body weight. As noted earlier, a professional athlete probably has a more favorable body composition—more muscle and less fat—than an inactive retired office worker, even though both are the same height and weight.

Weight, nevertheless, does play some part in body composition. A standard height and weight chart, however, usually provides a considerable range of so-called ideal weights for any given height. (See chart in Appendix B.) How you assess your weight according to the chart will depend to some extent on your body build. For example, the "ideal" weight of a woman 5 feet 5 inches may be anywhere from 111 to 142 pounds, depending on her body build. The smaller her body build, the closer her weight should be to the lower end of the range of desirable weights given for her height on the chart. The size of your wrist gives you a good idea of your body build. A woman 5 feet 5 inches whose wrist measures 5 inches around, for example, should be closer to 111 than to 142 pounds. You can use Table 1–7 to help you decide whether your body build is small, medium, or large.

While the "ideal" numbers in the familiar height and weight charts have their limitations, they may be of some use in assessing body composition. (They can at least confirm evidence based on subjective findings such as the mirror test, discussed below.) A weight much higher than average for your height may suggest problems in body composition, especially if you are relatively inactive. A steady increase in weight over the years since your mid-twenties or an increase in your waist measure-

---

Table 1–7

Determining Body Build

Measure the circumference of your wrist. The heading under which your measurement falls indicates your body build. All measurements are given in inches.

	Small	Medium	Large
Female	5.5" or less	5.6"–6.2"	6.3" or more
Male	6.7" or less	6.8"–7.4"	7.5" or more

ment are both fairly accurate indications that a disproportionate amount of the extra weight is likely to be in the form of fat, not muscle. In other words, your body fat percentage is probably high.

Because lean body tissue is denser than fat (muscle sinks, for example, while fat floats), underwater weighing is the most accurate means of assessing body composition. If the athlete and the retired office worker were weighed under water, the athlete would weigh more because the denser muscular tissue would displace more water than the less dense fatty tissue. Underwater weighing is not too convenient, so many fitness programs rely instead on skinfold calipers to assess body composition. This device measures the amount of fat lying just beneath the skin, where 50 percent of the body's fat is usually located. Mathematical equations convert the skinfold measurements into an estimate of total body fat.

If you have access to a physical fitness laboratory, you may be able to obtain a precise evaluation of body composition by using underwater weighing or skinfold measurement. Otherwise, like most people, you probably will have to rely on less exact but more practical procedures to find out your percentage of body fat.

Table 1–8 shows how one procedure for obtaining body fat percentages for females works. This technique, designed for women ages 17 to 26 and ages 27 to 50, requires a tape measure and a little arithmetic.

For males, there's a much simpler procedure for assessing body composition. Jack Wilmore, an exercise physiologist, has developed a formula for estimating the percentage of body fat for men based on waist girth and weight. Using Wilmore's data, Brian Sharkey, also an exercise physiologist, developed the self-assessment procedure illustrated in Table 1–9, below. Unfortunately, no similar test is available for women.

An easier way to estimate body composition—and it works for both men and women—is the pinch test described by Jean Mayer, an authority on overweight. Locate on your body a fold of skin and subcutaneous fat that may be lifted free—between the thumb and forefinger—from the underlying soft tissue and bone. Some of the body areas that can be used for this test are the back of the upper arm, the side of the lower chest, the back just below the shoulder blade, the back of the calf, or the abdomen. Once you've grasped the fold of skin, do your best to measure it. Mayer explains:

> In general, the layer beneath the skin should be between
> one-fourth and one-half inch; the skinfold is a double
> thickness and should therefore be one-half to one inch. A
> fold markedly greater than one inch—for example in the
> back of the arm—indicates excessive body fatness; one
> markedly thinner than one-half inch, abnormal thinness.

But the easiest test of all is the mirror test, which can help you estimate body fat. Mayer suggests that you simply look at yourself naked in a mirror. "If you *look* fat, you probably *are* fat," he notes.

31

Table 1–8

Test for Percentage of a Female's Body Fat

The arithmetical formulas to estimate the percentage of body fat are described in full in Appendix C, Tables 1 and 2.

Example of girth measurement for women ages 17 to 26

Measurement of abdomen (33 inches) converted into Constant A	44.12
Add measurement of right thigh (19 inches) converted into Constant B	+39.53
	83.65
Subtract measurement of right forearm (9 inches) converted into Constant C	−38.79
	44.86
Subtract 19.6*	−19.6
The result (rounded off) is 25 percent body fat.	25.26

Example of girth measurement for women ages 27 to 50

Measurement of abdomen (34.5 inches) converted into Constant A	40.97
Add measurement of right thigh (20.5 inches) converted into Constant B	+25.35
	66.32
Subtract measurement of right calf (12.5 inches) converted into Constant C	−18.08
	48.24
Subtract 18.4*	−18.4
The result (rounded off) is 30 percent body fat.	29.84

Assessing your body fat percentage. If your body fat percentage is more than 30 percent, consider yourself to be overfat. If your body fat percentage is more than 35 percent, consider yourself to be obese.

*For readers interested in an explanation of the numbers to be subtracted, see Frank I. Katch and William D. McArdle, "Evaluation of Body Composition," *Nutrition, Weight Control and Exercise,* Houghton Mifflin Company, 1977.

Table 1–9

Test for Percentage of a Male's Body Fat

A male whose weight and waist girth appear on the graph below can plot his body fat percentage. For example, a man who weighs 170 pounds with a 34-inch waist can establish that his body fat is about 18 percent.

Weight	Body fat percentage	Waist

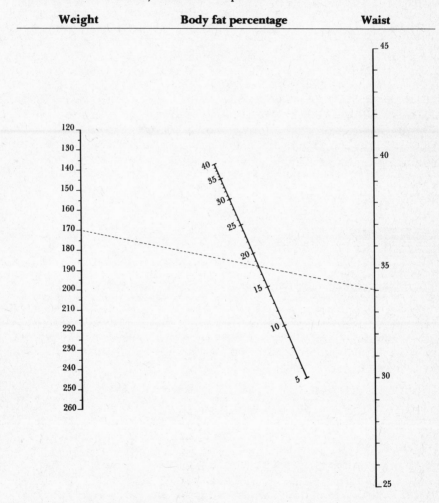

Assessing your body fat percentage. If your body fat percentage is between 20 and 25 percent, consider yourself to be overfat. If your body fat percentage is more than 25 percent, consider yourself to be obese.

33

Muscular strength

Your ability to lift a heavy suitcase or bag of groceries gives you a very rough idea of muscular strength. If you experience difficulty removing an ordinary lid from a jar, say, you may lack *minimal* muscular strength. To undertake an assessment of your precise muscular strength could mean comprehensive testing of the body's major muscle groups—a time-consuming process requiring expensive equipment that's not widely available. Such a procedure would be impractical as well as unnecessary for routine self-assessment. Instead, you can settle for a test of grip strength, involving a single muscle group but one that correlates well with tests of general body strength.

The most accurate way to test grip strength is by means of a hand dynamometer. You can usually locate one at a college gym, or even at some well-equipped high schools. To take the test, hold the dynamometer in one hand (preferably the hand you write with), squeeze the device as hard as you can, then read your score in pounds (or kilograms) on the dial. Consult Table 1–10 for an interpretation of your grip score.

If a hand dynamometer is not available, you can still determine whether you possess a minimum level of muscular strength by taking the self-tests described in Table 1–11. If you are able to carry out each of these

---

Table 1–10

Ratings for Grip Strength Dynamometer Test

The scores below are given in pounds. Because there is usually some change in body composition with increased age, scores should be adjusted to reflect an age-related decrease in the ratio of muscle to fat. People over age fifty should, therefore, add about 10 percent to their score. Example: If you are a woman fifty-one years old and you have a score of 49, then multiply 49 by 10 percent $(49 \times .10)$. The product is 4.9. Adding 4.9 to 49 gives an adjusted score of 53.9, which falls within the low rating.

	Very high	High	Moderate	Low	Very low
Female	Above 89	83–89	56–82	49–55	Below 49
Male	Above 154	136–154	105–135	91–104	Below 91

Assessing your grip strength score. If your score falls within the low or very low rating on the grip test, your overall muscular strength is probably also low or very low. If you choose to improve muscular strength by undertaking a specific exercise program, you are likely to see in time a dramatic improvement in your performance in activities requiring muscular strength. (See Chapter 5 for advice on planning an exercise program in this area.)

Table 1–11

Tests of Minimal Muscular Strength

All of the tests below can be looked on as pass-fail tests: Either you can do them or you can't. If you can do them, you probably have minimal muscular strength. (Most of these exercises are depicted in the Glossary of Exercises.)

Muscle group	Test	Directions	Passing score
Abdominals (Don't try if you have back trouble)	Sit-up (bent knees)	Start with lower back flat on floor and knees bent. Keep hands and arms in front. Bring head and shoulders from floor until you reach a sitting position. Do not push against floor with hands.	Do one sit-up without your feet being held down.
Back (Don't try if you have back trouble)	Back and hip extension	Lie face down with a pillow under your waist, hands clasped behind your neck, with legs and hips held down (you'll need someone to assist). Lift your head and shoulders from floor and hold for 10 seconds. With hands on floor and your upper body held down, lift legs with knees straight; hold yourself off the floor for 10 seconds.	Hold each of the movements for 10 seconds
Legs (Don't try if you have knee trouble)	Full deep-knee bend	Perform one full deep-knee bend and return to a standing position. Heels can leave the floor; arms extended forward may be helpful.	Perform one complete movement correctly
Shoulders, chest, and arms	Push-up*	Start in push-up position with arms straight, fingers forward. Lower chest to floor with back straight, then return to starting position.	Perform one complete movement correctly
Shoulders, chest, and arms	Front support*	Start in push-up position with arms straight, fingers forward. Over a 5-second period, lower chest to floor slowly with back straight.	Lower chest to floor over a 5-second period

*Men and women tend to differ in upper-body strength. While useful as a minimum standard for most men, it is not a fair test for most women (though some women do very well at push-ups).

35

simple tests, it would indicate that you have at least minimal muscular strength as measured by the capacity of a muscle group to lift or hold your own body weight. If your current activities include a good deal of pushing, pulling, and lifting, you probably can exceed the levels of strength measured in these tests. If you fall short of accomplishing one or more of the tests, which are only minimal measures, you may want to include development of muscular strength in your fitness program. Adequate muscular strength can help prevent muscle strain and low-back pain.

Muscular endurance

Somewhat dependent upon your level of muscular strength is your muscular endurance. For example, it takes a certain amount of strength

---

Table 1–12

Tests of Muscular Endurance

Follow the directions for the sit-up test; the purpose is to complete as many sit-ups in 60 seconds as possible. Follow the directions for the push-up or modified push-up test; the purpose is to complete as many push-ups as possible. (These exercises are depicted in the Glossary of Exercises.)

Muscle group	Test	Directions
Abdominals (Don't try if you have back trouble)	60-second sit-up (bent knees)	Start with your back flat on the floor and knees bent, feet flat on floor, hands clasped behind your neck. With feet held down (you'll need someone to assist), perform as many sit-ups as possible in 60 seconds. Touch elbows to your knees or thighs and return to the full starting position each time.
Shoulders, chest, and arms	Push-up*	Start in push-up position with arms straight, fingers forward. Lower chest to floor with back straight, then return to starting position. Your score is the maximum number of correct push-ups performed in succession.
Shoulders, chest, and arms	Modified push-up*	Same as in push-up, except that you support yourself with your knees, keeping your back straight.

---

*Many women may have insufficient strength to perform even a single push-up when using the push-up technique described above. The modified push-up allows such women to support themselves with their knees, thus reducing the need for upper-body strength in a test of muscular endurance.

36

to lift a suitcase, but it takes a certain amount of muscular endurance to hold it off the floor for five minutes. If your muscles usually feel sore a day or two after you weed, say, or shovel snow, or row a boat, you may be low in muscular endurance. If you tend to talk a lot about your "aching muscles," you may want to focus on improving your muscular endurance.

Sit-ups are commonly used to measure the muscular endurance of the abdominal muscles, and push-ups are used to measure the shoulders, chest, and arms. Following the directions in Table 1–12, see how many sit-ups you can do in sixty seconds and the number of consecutive push-ups you can complete correctly. Then compare your score with the ratings in Tables 1–13 and 1–14. These ratings are only estimates, but they can be useful in your self-assessment.

Table 1–13

Ratings for 60-Second Sit-Up Test

The scores below are for the number of sit-ups completed in 60 seconds. Ratings for scores are based on age and sex.

Age	Very high	High	Moderate	Low	Very low
Female					
15–29	Above 43	39–43	33–38	29–32	Below 29
30–39	Above 35	31–35	25–30	21–24	Below 21
40–49	Above 30	26–30	19–25	16–18	Below 16
50–59	Above 25	21–25	15–20	11–14	Below 11
60–69	Above 20	16–20	10–15	6–9	Below 6
Male					
15–29	Above 47	43–47	37–42	33–36	Below 33
30–39	Above 39	35–39	29–34	25–28	Below 25
40–49	Above 34	30–34	24–29	20–23	Below 20
50–59	Above 29	25–29	19–24	15–18	Below 15
60–69	Above 24	20–24	14–19	10–13	Below 10

Assessing your sit-up test score. This test measures muscular endurance of the abdominal muscles. A low or very low score can be improved by selecting weight training exercises for these muscles from the Glossary of Exercises.

Table 1–14

Ratings for Modified Push-Up and Push-Up Tests

The scores below are for the number of push-ups completed in succession. Ratings for scores are based on age and sex.

Age	Very high	High	Moderate	Low	Very low
Female (Modified push-up)					
15–29	Above 48	34–48	17–33	6–16	Below 6
30–39	Above 39	25–39	12–24	4–11	Below 4
40–49	Above 34	20–34	8–19	3–7	Below 3
50–59	Above 29	15–29	6–14	2–5	Below 2
60–69	Above 19	5–19	3–4	1–2	0
Male (Push-up)					
15–29	Above 54	45–54	35–44	20–34	Below 20
30–39	Above 44	35–44	25–34	15–24	Below 15
40–49	Above 39	30–39	20–29	12–19	Below 12
50–59	Above 34	25–34	15–24	8–14	Below 8
60–69	Above 29	20–29	10–19	5–9	Below 5

Assessing your push-up test score. This test evaluates the muscular endurance of your shoulder, arm, and chest muscles. A low or very low score can be improved by weight training exercises for these muscles from the Glossary of Exercises.

Flexibility

Flexibility—how limber you are—encompasses the ability to move a joint through its normal range of motion. To walk up a flight of stairs, for example, you need some flexibility in the hips, knees, and ankles.

Good trunk flexibility may help protect you against low-back pain, which can be related, in part, to tightness of the hamstring muscles (located in the back of the thighs), hips, and lower back. As with muscular strength and endurance, overall flexibility cannot be readily assessed by a single test. One measure of flexibility that can be particularly useful is described in Table 1–15, which shows you how to evaluate your ability to bend your trunk forward. Then check your ratings in Table 1–16.

Table 1–15

Test of Trunk Flexibility

Before beginning this test, do some warm-up stretching exercises, such as bending sideways, forward, and backward several times, and rotating your trunk. Warmups may not only make it easier to perform the test, they may also help prevent strain or injury. In doing this test and the warm-ups that precede it, make your movements slow and gradual—never fast or jerky. Once warmed up, follow the procedure described below to test your trunk flexibility.

Directions

1. Place on the floor a strip of adhesive tape about a foot or more in length. You will also need a yardstick.
2. Sit on the floor with your legs extended and your heels about 5 inches apart. Position yourself so that your heels reach the near edge of the adhesive tape.
3. Position the yardstick on the floor between your legs so that the 1-inch mark is at the end of the yardstick closest to your body and the 15-inch mark touches the near edge of the adhesive tape on which your heels are placed.
4. Slowly reach with both hands as far forward as possible. Touch your fingertips to the yardstick and hold this position momentarily. Check the yardstick and note the distance you've reached.
5. Try this three times. (Do not attempt to add length by jerking forward.) Your flexibility score is the best of the three trials.

Table 1–16

Ratings for Trunk Flexibility Test

The scores below are for the number of inches reached. Ratings for scores are based on sex.

	Very high	High	Moderate	Low	Very low
Female	Above 23	21–23	17–20	13–16	Below 13
Male	Above 21	19–21	14–18	12–13	Below 12

Assessing your trunk flexibility score. Women tend to be more flexible than men, as reflected in the scores listed in Table 1–16. If your score on the trunk flexibility test falls within the low or very low rating, you may wish to do regularly some of the various hamstring stretching exercises suggested in the Glossary of Exercises. No matter what you score on this test, keep in mind that flexibility involves more than just the lower back and hamstring muscles. Refer to Chapter 5 for other aspects of flexibility.

Table 1–17, below, summarizes the results of the self-assessment tests you've now completed. After you've checked the results, you may decide to consider setting some fitness goals for yourself.

Table 1–17

Fitness Assessment Summary

After completing the self-assessment tests, fill in the Table below to get a rough estimate of how you rate in each of the five components of physical fitness. For some tests, you will have a score and rating to record in the Results column. For others, you can simply note with a check mark that you completed a full deep-knee bend, say. The Comments column provides space for noting any areas that need improvement.

Begin Table 1–17 by filling in your activity index and estimated level of activity (see page 22).

Activity index:_____ **Estimated level of activity:**_____

Components	Tests	Results	Comments
Cardiorespiratory endurance	Modified step test	_____	_____
	Oxygen consumption (cardiac stress test)	_____ /	_____
Body composition	Percentage body fat (female)	_____	_____
	Percentage body fat (male)	_____	_____
	Pinch test	_____	_____
	Mirror test	_____	_____
Muscular strength	Grip strength	_____	_____
	Sit-up	_____	_____
	Back and hip extension	_____	_____
	Full deep-knee bend	_____	_____
	Push-up	_____	_____
	Front support	_____	_____

Components	Tests	Results	Comments
Muscular endurance	60-second sit-up	_____	_____
	Push-up	_____	_____
	Modified push-up	_____	_____
Flexibility	Trunk flexibility	_____	_____

Setting goals

With the fitness assessment summary now completed, you may want to set yourself only a general goal—to promote your overall physical fitness by concentrating on the particular components that seem to be most in need of improvement. Or, like many of the readers of *Consumer Reports* we heard from, you may want to cope with a specific health problem or achieve a specific fitness goal.

For the sake of your health you may find you need to improve the way your heart and lungs function. Perhaps you decide it's time to lose weight and tone up some muscles to enhance your appearance. Or you may believe it prudent to keep limber to protect yourself from disabling stiffness in your later years. These goals, of course, are all keyed to specific components of physical fitness. To fortify heart and lungs, you work on cardiorespiratory endurance. To slim down and firm up, you concentrate on body composition. To be limber, you work on flexibility.

What if you want to get in shape for tennis, increase your stamina, or improve your posture? The appropriate exercise regimen to achieve such goals may not be as clearly keyed to a single component: It may require a combination of more than one component. For example, getting in shape for tennis calls for developing CRE, increasing the strength and muscular endurance of your arms and legs, and improving flexibility.

No matter which approaches to fitness you favor, you may find it helpful to look over Table 1–18. It lists the twenty-nine goals cited most often by our *Consumer Reports* respondents together with the fitness components most likely to be strengthened by a program designed to meet each of the goals.

Many common fitness goals, as Table 1–18 indicates, depend for their realization on simultaneously upgrading more than one fitness component. But even if you choose to work on just a single component, such a program would still be likely to improve other components as well. For instance, jogging undertaken primarily to improve your cardiorespiratory condition will probably also improve your body composition and have some effect on the muscular endurance of your legs.

Cardiorespiratory endurance ratings, body fat percentages, and grip

41

test scores tend to be abstract and impersonal concepts. Few of the *Consumer Reports* readers who wrote to us about fitness used terms such as increased CRE or improved body composition to describe their goals. What many hoped for from a fitness regimen was "freedom from back-aches," "more stamina," "better muscle tone," and the like.* Such goals are readily translatable into fitness components. For example, as noted earlier, an increase in muscular strength and flexibility, especially in the muscles and joints of the lower trunk, could help reduce susceptibility to low-back pain.

Once you have completed the fitness assessment summary, reviewed Table 1–18 for ideas about goals you might like to achieve, and noted which components are most involved in achieving those goals, then you will have a better sense of the specific training program you may want to pursue. Refer to the contents page for the chapters that are most relevant to your goals.

Improvement in physical fitness may not be the only achievement of those who set fitness goals for themselves. Many *Consumer Reports* readers who wrote about their own current fitness programs mentioned intangible by-products of various forms of exercise. An eighteen-year-old, L.R. of Dallas, Texas, for example, believes a program of regular jogging has given her "a sense of peace and calm as well as a feeling of personal accomplishment."

Running every day, according to T.C., age thirty, a Massachusetts clinical psychologist, "is guaranteed to relax me and clear my mind of any disturbing thoughts. It is almost a form of psychotherapy." P.E., age twenty-nine, of Redwood, California, says that by pushing herself beyond what she thought she could endure, her exercise program has given her "a whole new image" of herself.

A good number of such testimonials turned up in hundreds of letters from *Consumer Reports* readers. Many of them say that since undertaking a regular fitness regimen, they sleep better, eat more sensibly, work harder. Many say they have greater enthusiasm, feel better about themselves, and are less jittery or irritable; quite a few say their sex life has improved. These positive side effects of improved physical fitness are difficult to explain, and they are harder to predict than improvement in the mea-surable components. Although no one can guarantee that becoming physically fit by following an exercise program will enhance the quality of life, virtually all of CU's respondents thought it did.

What physical fitness training can do is make some distinct, measur-able improvements in one or more of the five components. These in turn

---

*Some *Consumer Reports* readers told us that enhanced fitness helped relieve the discomfort of varicose veins or emphysema. Their letters reflect their conviction that exercise helped ease their symptoms. These are only anecdotal reports, of course.

can help you achieve some of the fitness goals you have set for yourself. Success can't be guaranteed, and it certainly isn't easy to achieve in any case. But for many people, physical fitness is definitely worth a try. And trying for it can even be fun.

Table 1–18

Specific Fitness Goals and Components Involved in Their Achievement

Goals	CRE	Body composition	Muscular strength	Muscular endurance	Flexibility
Recuperate from surgery	✓		✓	✓	✓
Rehabilitation after a stroke	✓		✓	✓	✓
Prevent, eliminate, or reduce low-back pain; recover from an orthopedic problem			✓	✓	✓
Make pregnancy and childbirth easier	✓		✓	✓	✓
Eliminate or reduce breathlessness brought on by climbing stairs, etc.	✓	✓		✓	
Increase stamina in such activities as jogging, swimming, dancing, bicycling, long walks	✓	✓		✓	
Increase resistance to muscle fatigue	✓		✓	✓	
Increase muscular effectiveness for daily tasks, sports activities			✓	✓	✓
Become more muscular; firm up muscle tone		✓	✓	✓	
Rehabilitation after a heart attack	✓	✓			
Reduce risk of circulatory and respiratory system disorders	✓	✓			
Lower high blood pressure	✓	✓			
Help to improve control of diabetes	✓	✓			
Lower cholesterol and/or triglyceride levels	✓	✓			
Increase high density lipoprotein cholesterol	✓	✓			
Reduce discomfort from arthritis			✓		✓
Prevent, eliminate, or reduce muscle and/or joint injury			✓		✓
Decrease muscle soreness due to physical activity				✓	✓

43

Goals	CRE	Body composition	Muscular strength	Muscular endurance	Flexibility
Have more energy at the end of a day's activities	✔			✔	
Improve posture				✔	✔
Reduce menstrual discomfort			✔		✔
Survive a heart attack	✔				
Lower the resting heart rate	✔				
Reduce asthmatic discomfort during exercise	✔				
Increase range of movement and become more limber					✔
Reduce discomfort from tension					✔
Improve fit of clothes		✔			
Lose weight or gain weight		✔			
Look trimmer by reducing the girth of waist, hips, thighs, arms		✔			

2

Physical Fitness Training Principles

The human body has an extraordinary ability to respond to the physical demands placed on it if sound training principles are used and the level of demands is escalated slowly. In a graduated program, the muscles involved progressively increase in strength and endurance with each small increment of activity. As the individual muscle fibers increase in size, the muscles gain in strength. This process, known as *hypertrophy,* occurs slowly as the demands on muscles gradually increase. Abrupt increases in activity levels, however, could cause tendon and muscle injuries.

Progressive overload

If you have never lifted anything heavier than a ten-pound bag of groceries, you may not find it so easy to pick up a neighbor's thirty-pound child, let alone carry the toddler in your arms. But the parents of the child would probably not find it difficult. Undoubtedly, they have become quite accustomed to carrying that thirty-pound child about. The weight would be less of a strain for them because they had been lifting the youngster almost daily since the child was born. Or suppose you have a stockroom job that requires you to stack fifty-pound packages. If you had to switch to stacking seventy-pound packages, it would probably give you some difficulty at first, but over a few weeks your body would adjust to the heavier work load.

When you make demands such as these on your body, its first response is to mobilize its resources to accomplish the greater work load. The muscles involved will strain somewhat to accomplish the task; heart rate, breathing, and blood flow to those muscles will all increase sharply. But with repetition of the activity over a period of time, the body becomes adapted to the increased work load. The heart, lungs, and muscles function more efficiently, accomplishing the same work with less exertion.

45

This kind of experience—adaptation of the body to new demands—results from *progressive overload,* the first of two fundamental principles of sound fitness training. (The second, *specificity,* is discussed on page 47.) Progressive overload can be achieved by increasing one or more of three factors: intensity, duration, and frequency. To lift heavier packages in a stockroom job means that the *intensity* of the activity has increased. If you also put in overtime, you increase the *duration.* And working six days a week instead of five increases the *frequency.* As your body adapts to the new demands, you acquire a new level of competence and comfort. Last week's exertion becomes today's comfortable work load. Of course, if you reduce your level of activity, the opposite occurs: Your body adjusts to a lower level of competency and strength, and yesterday's acceptable work load becomes next week's overload.

If you ever had an arm or a leg in a cast or been confined to bed after surgery, you no doubt recall how your body adapted to the lack of movement. The size and strength of the affected muscles dwindled and there was a general decline in strength, endurance, and flexibility. As you recovered, you probably applied progressive overload even if you didn't have professional guidance for your rehabilitation. When the cast was removed or when strict bed rest was no longer necessary, you most likely arranged your day so that you would avoid any excessive effort. Perhaps you limited your stair climbing to once a day, took a nap after lunch, and went to bed early in the evening. When you returned to your regular routine, it was probably only part time at first. Gradually you extended the range of your activities until eventually you were able to resume everything you had formerly been able to do.

Your recovery was geared to a slow but steady restoration of impaired muscular strength, endurance, and flexibility. By progressively demanding more and more from your body, you made use of your body's normal ability to adapt in time to new demands. Sound physical fitness programs, like therapeutic programs, are based on the body's self-protective capacity for adaptation. If you start with a work load at, or only slightly above, your ordinary level of fitness and then very slowly and steadily increase the work load, you will make slow but steady improvement in your fitness level.

The positive adaptations your body makes to new and increasingly rigorous demands are known as *training effects.* For example, the training effects of a program for cardiorespiratory endurance (CRE) would include reduced heart rates while at rest and during activity and also breathing more comfortably during activity. The training effects of a program to improve body composition would include an increase in the size and weight of skeletal muscles and a decrease in body fat. In short, training effects are the benefits you get from a regular exercise program, practiced in accordance with the training principle of progressive overload.

When overloading becomes excessive, however, there may be unpleasant and even painful reactions. Starting out at too demanding a level of activity or going too soon to the next level usually results in aches, pains, and discouragement.

If you experience symptoms such as the following, the cause is probably excessive overload:

■ Rapid heart rate—at the level experienced during the activity—persisting five to ten minutes after the activity has stopped.

■ Fatigue continuing twenty-four hours after the activity has stopped.

■ Muscle soreness (charley horse or feeling muscle-bound).

If you gradually increase the demands you make on yourself when you begin a fitness program, you can avoid problems such as these. A little overload goes a long way. The watchword should be, "Train, don't strain." Start with a slight overload and increase it steadily to get your training effects with little or no discomfort.

Specificity

Hand in hand with progressive overload goes *specificity*, the second fundamental principle of sound fitness training. Your fitness program must be specifically designed to meet your goals. You need quite different programs to get in shape for varsity basketball than you do for weekend tennis doubles. Exercises to develop arm strength aren't the same as those used for rehabilitation after a heart attack.

Sometimes, of course, an exercise program may be inappropriate for a particular goal. Take, for example, E.S., a thirty-three-year-old from Chicago. "Throughout most of my life, I've been rather heavy around the middle," E.S. wrote. He described himself as 5 feet 8 inches, with a 40-inch waist when he first turned to exercise. At a friend's suggestion, E.S. did "lots of sit-ups—morning, noon, and night" for three months. Even though he was doing hundreds a day, his waist size didn't change and he finally gave up. However, a month or so later, he "read that aerobic activities like running or cycling are supposed to be excellent for weight loss. I took up cycling, riding an hour a day, five days a week, and attempted to control my eating. After a few months I had to add some new notches to my belt—down to a 38." A year later, he reported, he had a 34-inch waist.

For every fitness goal there is a variety of appropriate activities to choose from. Your choice should take into consideration such factors as how an activity is paced, the level of skill and fitness prerequisite required, intensity, duration, and frequency (see below). Other aspects to consider—the degree of sociality involved in an activity, its convenience, its cost, your current level of health, your age, and your interests—are covered in Chapter 6.

How an activity is paced. This can be an important consideration. If it is up to you to set the pace, there may be no problem: You can go at your own rate. But if others are involved, your benefit from an activity can be affected. You will need to consider, say, other participants' skill levels, the demands of an activity leader, or the need to keep up with other participants.

Level of skill and fitness prerequisite. If your activity index (see page 22) is low or if you performed poorly in one or two of the self-assessment tests in Chapter 1, you should choose activities that are self-paced and appropriate for your particular level of fitness. Some activities require such complex skills or such a high level of fitness that they may not be practical for anyone beginning a fitness program. Be sure to choose activities that you can perform with enough skill to achieve the goals you have set for yourself. You do not need to have athletic skills, for example, to improve your CRE with a jogging program. But to improve CRE by playing tennis, you need enough skill to sustain a volley long enough to achieve and maintain an elevated heart rate.

Designing an exercise program

Below are some general guidelines to help you decide on a suitable exercise program. Detailed information about various exercise programs and activities are found in Chapters 7 and 8. Whatever your fitness goals and whatever your choice of exercise, the cornerstones of your program will be progressive overload and specificity.

By making use of the information in Chapters 7 and 8 to help you select an activity to achieve a particular goal, you are applying the principle of specificity. You may find yourself juggling variables and weighing personal priorities as you consider all the criteria before you make your choice. For example, you may end up selecting an activity not so much because it's interesting and enjoyable but because it's convenient. Fortunately, no selection need be permanent. You can always change activities to meet changing needs and interests. (And that is a good reason to avoid making too great a financial commitment at the beginning of a fitness program.)

Once you have decided on an appropriate exercise program, you should begin to apply the principle of progressive overload. Ask yourself three questions: How hard should I exercise? How long should I keep at it in each session? How often should I do it? In other words, you need to attain training effects by adjusting the intensity, duration, and frequency of your exercise sessions.

How hard? The *intensity* at which you start a specific program depends on how fit you are. But no matter what your current level of fitness, improvement will come only as your body adapts to the increased demands you place on it. Suppose you swim one lap of a 25-yard pool in one minute but you need to rest for two minutes before you can swim another lap. That effort would represent your beginning level of intensity. Then suppose your program calls for swimming every other day. After a few weeks, you will find you can swim the first lap faster and begin the second lap after a shorter rest period. What has happened is that you have increased your intensity (faster lap time and shorter rest period) as your body responds to the new demands placed on it.

Similarly, if you are a jogger beginning an exercise program to improve CRE, you could increase intensity by quickening your pace or by running uphill. If you are riding a stationary bicycle to improve body composition, you can intensify your effort by increasing the resistance against which you pedal or by pedaling faster. If you are a weight trainer working for muscular strength and endurance, you can put more weight on the bar or increase the number of repetitions. If you are doing calisthenics to increase flexibility, you could raise the intensity by stretching farther.

In establishing your beginning level of intensity, always remember it is best to be conservative. You should not feel that you are working hard when you exercise. Be patient; you can increase your work load gradually as your body becomes conditioned. During CRE activity, your heart rate serves as your guide to how fast you should increase your work load. During muscular strength and muscular endurance training, it will be the amount of resistance or the number of repetitions you can manage. In flexibility workouts, the extent of your stretch will be the criterion.

How long? The *duration* of your exercise session will depend in part on its intensity. The less demanding the activity, the longer the session can be. If you jog, you could run for a longer time by slowing your pace or you could run for a shorter time at a faster pace. In weight training, if you increase the load, you will probably have to reduce the number of repetitions until you adapt to the greater weight.

But when you have limited time for exercise it can be useful to increase the intensity to make the most of the time available. A good tennis player, for example, will get more training effects from forty-five minutes of vigorous singles with an equally skilled opponent than from two hours of doubles against less skilled competitors.

Because intensity and duration are so closely related, you will often have to adjust one to the other. For example, high-intensity activity will usually be limited in duration because fatigue sets in more quickly. If you want to work at high intensity, you can compensate for this to some extent by using a method of training called *interval training*. It involves alternating brief rest periods with bouts of exercise. A jogger might alternate one minute of walking with two minutes of jogging. A rope skipper might break a session with a one-minute rest period every two minutes or with two-minute intervals of reduced intensity—stretching exercises, say, or calisthenics. A swimmer might take a rest from the crawl by doing the sidestroke for a lap or two. To increase training effects with interval training, you can shorten the resting period or step up the intensity.

How often? The *frequency* of your workouts depends on such factors as how much time you have available, your goals, and the time span in which you hope to achieve them. Remember that physical fitness is only temporary. You may begin to lose some training effects as soon as two or three days after a workout. Obviously, then, weekend exercise is not enough. Daily workouts may be somewhat more beneficial than a session every other day, but for a general fitness program, an every-other-day schedule seems to offer the best return for the time invested. If weight loss is a goal, you will probably need five or more exercise periods a week to use up the calories your program calls for. Whatever your fitness goals, however, once you have achieved your desired fitness level, you can probably maintain it with fewer exercise periods a week.

Table 2–1 illustrates how the training principles of specificity and progressive overload can be used to increase fitness levels for each of the five components.

How to get started

If your current level of activity is low, you should start out very slowly. Begin at a starting level of one of the model programs (see Chapter 7). Don't step up the pace until you find that your muscles have adjusted to the new demands placed on them, and even then progress should be slow. You may decide to begin with a model walking or jogging program. After several weeks or more on the model program, you may wish to switch to one of the activities described in Chapter 8. Or you may want to experiment with a mix of several different activities once you have moved beyond the initial stage of conditioning.

No matter which activity you select, it should always be preceded and followed by warm-up and cool-down routines (see stretching model program in Chapter 7). Plan to give at least ten minutes to warming up, including stretching, before you begin a workout. And cool down or recover by tapering off your exercise for at least five minutes after the workout.

No matter how pressed you are for time, don't skip the warm-up period. It serves several important functions. It can prevent or reduce muscle and joint injuries and soreness. If you are working on improving CRE, a warm-up period can prepare your cardiorespiratory system gradually for the high level of stress that exercise may place on it. And it can help you get psychologically ready for your exercise session.

Table 2–1

Application of Training Principles to Fitness Components

To benefit one or more of the five components of physical fitness, an activity must take into account the two fundamental training principles. To illustrate specificity, a sample of appropriate activities for each component is listed below. To define progressive overload, the requirements of intensity, duration, and frequency are given for each of the components. Note that for muscular endurance two approaches are offered: calisthenics and weight training; intensity and duration differ for the two.

Fitness components	Examples of specificity	Progressive overload		
		Intensity	Duration	Frequency
Cardiorespiratory endurance (see Chapter 3)	Bicycling, jogging, rope skipping, swimming, walking	Increase pace as heart rate permits; maintain heart rate in EBZ (see page 62)	Gradually prolong exercise time; 15 minutes is minimum for training effects	At least every other day
Body composition (see Chapter 4)	Bicycling, jogging, swimming, walking	Increase pace as heart rate permits; maintain heart rate in EBZ (see page 62)	Gradually prolong exercise time; 30 minutes is minimum for training effects	At least every other day; aim for 5 days a week if goal is to reduce body fat and/or weight
Muscular strength (see Chapter 5)	Weight training	Use barbells to perform 6 repetitions; at 10 repetitions, increase weight	Increase by repeating each set of 6–10 repetitions	At least every other day
Muscular endurance (see Chapter 5)	Calisthenics	Increase difficulty of exercises	Increase by repeating each set of repetitions	At least every other day
	Weight training	Use barbells to perform 15–25 repetitions; at 25 repetitions, increase weight	Increase by repeating each set of 15–25 repetitions	At least every other day
Flexibility (see Chapter 5)	Calisthenics, modern dance, yoga	Use moderate force to stretch joints	Gradually prolong stretching time for each exercise from 10 up to 60 seconds	At least every other day

Stretching—which should be a slow, easy, gradual process—can be particularly useful as a prelude to such activities as walking and jogging, which require the constant repetition of a limited range of motion of the hamstring, calf, and low-back muscles. Unless stretched, these muscles may tighten and thus cause a variety of discomforts and problems that could put a temporary—or even permanent—end to exercise.

The cool-down period, as the term implies, is a time of reduced activity at the end of a workout. If you have been running, for example, you would reduce the intensity of your activity by slowing to a walk for the last quarter-mile or so. During the cool-down period, your body returns to normal, with heart rate, breathing, and circulation all restored to near pre-exercise levels. With a cool-down period you are less likely to suffer nausea or lightheadedness, which can sometimes occur after strenuous exercise. Some people like to repeat the stretching exercises once over lightly as part of the cool-down, and they should now seem much easier and more relaxing than before the workout. Stretching out again at the end of the workout is a good way to prevent muscle tightness and cramping.

In Chapters 6 and 7, we offer suggestions about how best to launch an exercise program. We also suggest various strategies to help you keep going should some of your enthusiasm for exercise begin to fade.

Overenthusiasm can also be a problem. Crash exercising is something like crash dieting: In an excess of zeal or despair—or perhaps some of each—people set impossible goals and go overboard in an effort to achieve them. Instant fitness cannot be achieved, and in the aftermath, people often become so discouraged they lapse into a condition even worse than the one they were in before the crash program. But if you set realistic goals, select activities that can help you achieve them, and work gradually and steadily, you are likely to succeed.

3

Cardiorespiratory Endurance

Almost anywhere nowadays you're likely to see people running—in track shorts or sweat suits, alone or in pairs or in packs, on roads or sidewalks or cinderpaths. Some smile, some chat with each other, and some grimly chug ahead. They come in all ages and sizes. Among the *Consumer Reports* readers who wrote us about how they exercise, those on the road—the runners, joggers, and walkers—outnumbered those who exercise by bicycling, rope skipping, and swimming, All these activities are effective ways to achieve cardiorespiratory endurance (CRE).

Included in the large and diverse group of exercisers who wrote to *Consumer Reports* was seventy-six-year-old C.J. of Cleveland, who runs 600 to 700 steps in place every other day and walks an eighteen-hole golf course three times a week. Fifty-year-old R.P. of Downers Grove, Illinois, swims three to four times a week at the "Y"; she says her thirty-minute sessions in the pool firm up her body. And H.K. of Erie, Pennsylvania, a forty-four-year-old woman, dances on roller skates for four-hour periods three times a week.

For some *Consumer Reports* respondents, exercise is more than just a routine. N.B. of Lathrup Village, Missouri, wrote, "I have almost reached the point where I psychologically need the daily run." One thirty-year-old woman reported that her ballet classes "relieve all tensions of the day." F.G. of Conrad, Montana, said, "I started by walking to work and back. . . . Then I became addicted. . . . Even in six inches of snow and thirty below."

Such zeal is, of course, not universal; but deep enjoyment is widespread. W.H., forty-two, of Temple, Texas, for example, told Consumers Union, "The hour a day I spend running is the best part of my day." And A.D., forty-one, of Holland, Michigan, wrote that running provided "a refreshing oasis in a superficial, flashy, stroking, image-seeking society."

Some *Consumer Reports* readers take another path. They measure out their miles with little or no enjoyment, running only because they think they should. P.V., seventy, of New York City, found it "a terrible bore." Nevertheless, she expects to "keep running for another ten years," because otherwise she fears she would "melt away in a chair." Similarly, R.T., thirty-six, of San Juan, Puerto Rico, wrote, "I force myself to keep going year after year. . . . I jog at 6 AM, before I am awake enough to realize how much I hate it."

Love it, like it, or loathe it, these people spend hour after hour exercising out of a deep conviction that it will benefit them. Many said that they began exercising to overcome their lack of stamina. Most reported that they achieved good results. They told Consumers Union that their energy levels have increased, they are sleeping better, feel more relaxed, suffer fewer headaches, have less insomnia, and get fewer colds than they did before they started exercising. They smoke less, drink less, and control their weight more easily. Quite a few reported a better sex life. Although it is difficult to prove that exercise caused all the good results, many of the reported benefits of regular training are consistent with increased CRE.

In Chapter 1 we defined CRE as the ability to perform moderately strenuous activity over a long period of time at less than maximum effort—to swim continuously for twenty minutes, say, or to walk two miles in a half hour. The terms CRE and aerobic fitness can be used interchangeably. Running a mile depends primarily on aerobic fitness—the ability of the cardiorespiratory system to deliver the regular, steady supply of oxygen required by the heart and other muscles.

An *aerobic* activity is any sustained, moderately strenuous effort carried on at an intensity level just high enough to let the heart and lungs keep pace with the increased need for oxygen required by the working muscles.

Sudden rigorous activity, such as sprinting—for a bus or a touchdown—is usually *anaerobic*. In other words, the intense burst of muscle activity outstrips the ability of the heart and lungs to step up the supply of oxygen needed during the sprint. Such maximum effort may leave you exhausted and gasping once the bus is boarded or the touchdown scored. When you're out of breath, you're out of oxygen. For several minutes after the anaerobic activity is ended, your heart and lungs work overtime to provide the oxygen needed to repay your "oxygen debt."

A 100-yard dash is almost purely anaerobic. A marathon is almost entirely aerobic. Most exercise, however, combines aerobic activity with anaerobic spurts. A mile run, for example, is mainly aerobic. But in the home stretch, the miler calls upon anaerobic reserves to surge ahead, take the lead, and fend off challengers; at the finish line, the miler is gasping for oxygen.*

---

*For more about oxygen and energy production, see Appendix D.

Anaerobic activity, such as sprinting, can be tolerated for only short periods of time. If your anaerobic reserves come into play at a relatively low level of activity and you become fatigued and exhausted easily, you probably have low CRE and low aerobic capacity. If your CRE is sufficient to sustain a high level of activity, then you probably have high aerobic capacity as well as high CRE. *Aerobic capacity* is the maximum amount of oxygen your cardiorespiratory system can deliver to the muscles during the most strenuous activity you can do.

You can increase your aerobic capacity by undertaking a regular CRE training program. How much you can improve depends on such things as your age, initial level of fitness, and the intensity, duration, and frequency of the training program you select. (To benefit CRE, an exercise must involve the body's largest muscle groups—the legs, including thighs, and the back.) For competitive athletes, there seems to be an inherent limit in aerobic capacity that they encounter within two years after beginning CRE training.* (Reaching a plateau on various occasions during training is also common and should not be confused with reaching a built-in limit.)

Cardiorespiratory training effects

W.D. of White Plains, New York, a woman of forty-eight, began a walking/jogging program to help her keep up with her family on hikes. At first, she told Consumers Union, walking a mile exhausted her. After several weeks she was able to alternate her walking with intervals of slow jogging. Soon she was doing more jogging, with intervals of walking. After two months, she could jog two miles with only brief walking intervals. Then she stalled. Weeks went by without any improvement. She wondered whether she would ever be able to jog the entire two-mile distance without having to walk at all. Finally it happened, during her fifth month on the program. "We were jogging on a nearby quarter-mile track, talking as usual," she reported, "when I suddenly realized that we were finishing the sixth lap and I hadn't walked yet." She wasn't panting and her heart wasn't pounding.

---

*Despite this limit, athletes can continue to improve their performance in long-distance events. They can often better their previous records by performing for longer periods of time at a greater percentage of their aerobic capacity. For example, long-distance runners who have reached their inherent limit and therefore cannot expect any further increase in aerobic capacity may still become capable of improving their time in running a race. Further CRE training may enable them to maintain a pace in running a marathon, for example, at a higher percentage of aerobic capacity for a longer period during the race. Indeed, some champion-class marathoners can run at more than 80 percent of their aerobic capacity for a full twenty-six miles—a feat that results in improved competitive time.

The cardiorespiratory endurance of the White Plains jogger had improved enough to increase her aerobic capacity significantly. The change had come from improvements in many elements of her cardio-respiratory system. The heart of the matter, of course, is the heart itself, the body's pump. The adult heart contracts from 50 to 100 times a minute with an average of 70 contractions per minute, depending on such factors as sex (6 to 8 beats higher in women), and occupation. The number of systoles (heart contractions) per minute is defined as the *heart rate*. The amount of blood pumped out of the heart by each systole is called the *stroke volume,* which varies in normal adults from 70 to 100 milliliters at rest. The stroke volume is usually larger in a slower beating heart, because a slow heart rate allows more time between beats (the diastolic time interval) for the heart to fill with blood. *Cardiac output* is the total amount of blood the heart pumps in one minute. It is computed by multiplying stroke volume by heart rate.

There was no documentation of the White Plains jogger's marked improvement in physical fitness. Her heart rate had not been checked and her stroke volume and cardiac output had not been estimated at the beginning of her training program and again when she had achieved her two-mile running goal. Nor had she been weighed and measured and some of her blood chemistries studied. The improvement was real, never-theless, and reflects specific training effects—positive adaptations of her body to progressively increasing demands. These included an increase in the size and strength of the heart muscle, a reduction in heart rate both at rest and during activity, an increase in stroke volume and cardiac output, and a reduction in the time it takes for the heart to return to resting levels after exercise.

At one time there was concern about "athlete's heart," an enlarged heart shadow found on chest X rays of some athletes. It was thought that a heart of greater than normal size and volume was synonymous with a heart enlarged by disease; therefore many athletes with such X rays were told to curtail their activities. It is now understood that athlete's heart—an enlarged heart shadow on chest X rays—is due to the increased size of the ventricular chamber as well as increased development of the heart muscle.* And muscular development is a beneficial training effect of a CRE program, resulting in a strengthened heart with a slow beat.

Other CRE training effects are an increase in the body's blood volume (the total amount of blood) and in plasma volume (plasma is the

---

*An enlarged heart shadow on chest X rays can take several shapes, only one of which represents the so-called athlete's heart. When doubt exists about whether an enlarged heart shadow warrants further examination—even after the chest X rays have been viewed by an experienced radiologist—additional testing, such as an electrocardiogram or echocardiogram, may be necessary.

fluid in which blood cells are carried). The larger total blood volume reflects a small increase in the number of red cells, which results in an improved oxygen-carrying capacity. The increase in blood plasma makes the blood less thick, enabling it to flow more easily and rapidly through the circulatory system.

People with hypertension (high blood pressure) may expect some improvement in resting blood pressure measurements as a result of CRE training. During active exercise, everyone's blood pressure, nonhypertensives and hypertensives alike, temporarily goes up because of more forceful and rapid heart contractions—a normal response to exercise. After the activity is over, blood pressure returns to resting levels. The less time it takes, the better shape you are in.

CRE training may also reduce some people's blood cholesterol levels. High cholesterol levels have been found to be associated with an increased risk of coronary heart disease. (The evidence relating this to increased blood triglycerides, another body fat, is not nearly as convincing.) Recent research has shown that the relationship between cholesterol and exercise is more complex than once thought. The portion of blood cholesterol associated with high density lipoproteins (HDL) actually is protective against coronary heart disease, while the opposite is true of low density lipoproteins. Levels of HDL cholesterol have been found to be higher in people who regularly do CRE exercises than in those who don't.

It also has been shown that the blood of well-trained athletes has a decreased tendency to clot, thereby theoretically diminishing the possibility of heart attack. The exact role of exercise in preventing coronary heart disease, however, is not clear. Various population studies suggest that there are fewer heart attacks and sudden deaths from heart attack among physically active people than sedentary people. But it is difficult to tell whether active people live longer because their activity makes them healthier, or whether they live longer and are more active because they are healthier to begin with. None of the studies is conclusive, although some of them—including the renowned Framingham study, which has followed almost the entire community of Framingham, Massachusetts, for more than thirty years—have identified factors that do seem to be closely associated with an increased risk of coronary heart disease. These factors include hypertension, elevated blood cholesterol, diabetes, and a sedentary life-style—all of which can be improved by regular CRE exercise.

For these reasons, then, some authorities are convinced that exercises such as the model programs for CRE described in Chapter 7 can help to avert coronary heart disease and help to rehabilitate heart attack victims. In coronary heart disease, the coronary arteries (the blood vessels that supply the heart muscle with blood containing oxygen and nutrients) become narrowed by deposits of cholesterol. This process, called atherosclerosis, takes place slowly, over a long period of time, and in some cases begins as early as young adulthood. Convincing evidence of coronary

57

artery atherosclerosis came from autopsies of young American soldiers killed in Korea and Vietnam. As the arteries continue to narrow, less blood can flow through them to nourish the heart muscle. When the coronary arteries can no longer supply the heart muscle with oxygen, that portion of the heart nourished by the affected arteries dies (a condition known as myocardial infarction).

If the area of heart muscle affected is not large, and if collateral (substitute) blood vessels from adjacent areas can take over and begin to nourish the affected portion, death from myocardial infarction may be prevented. Studies of animals show that exercise to enhance CRE can help develop these collateral blood vessels. Relatively little research has been done on human collateral circulation, but some investigators recommend exercise for persons with impaired coronary circulation more to promote the development of collateral blood vessels than to prevent progress of coronary heart disease itself.

T.B., a sixty-one-year-old *Consumer Reports* reader from Lansing, Michigan, is typical of a growing number of coronary heart disease victims whose recovery has been helped by exercise. Eight years earlier, because of severe chest pains, T.B. had tests that showed there was blockage of a coronary artery. Given a choice between a coronary bypass operation and an exercise program to try to build up his collateral circulation, T.B. chose exercise. In the beginning, he was in such poor shape that he had chest pain with the slightest exertion. He started a regimen that included prescribed coronary medication and a carefully controlled program of exercise on a stationary bicycle. His progress was slow but steady: After seven years he had improved enough to begin a jogging program. Again he began slowly and modestly, with half-mile outings that included two or three walking intervals. A year later he was regularly jogging twenty miles a week, without any walking breaks, and he told Consumers Union that he hoped soon to be doing four six-mile runs a week. His cardiologist finds his progress "unbelievable," and T.B. agrees: "I'm in better physical condition than the average person without a cardiac problem who is not a regular exerciser."

T.B. is an unusual example. Still, most cardiologists now recommend a gradual increase in exercise for people recovering from a heart attack or from heart surgery, and for people who may be at risk of heart attack. Such exercise programs must be approved by a physician and are usually carried out in a well-supervised facility.

Cardiac stress test

If a review of the medical guidelines in Chapter 1 left you with no doubts about your ability to handle an increase in activity, you will probably not need a cardiac stress test. For some, however, medical clearance and even a stress test are wise precautions. Among screening tests for coronary heart disease, a cardiac stress test (also known as an exercise tolerance test or treadmill test) is currently the simplest and cheapest available. The cost is usually $100 to $250.

Consumers Union's medical consultants believe that it is probably a good idea to discuss taking a stress test with your physician if you are over thirty-five and are considering a fitness program. A stress test is necessary if you have ever had coronary heart disease, have a family history of early-onset coronary heart disease, have diabetes or hypertension, smoke cigarettes, are being treated for high cholesterol, are more than twenty pounds overweight, or are accustomed to a sedentary life-style. How reliable the stress test is as a predictive tool, however, varies directly with the number of heart disease risk factors you have. For example, the stress test has proved to be of more value for detecting coronary heart disease in people who have hypertension and who smoke than for nonsmokers with normal blood pressure.*

If your physician agrees that you should take a cardiac stress test and suggests a convenient facility to take it in, Consumers Union's medical consultants recommend that you check out the facility—either with your physician or with the facility itself. The criteria to consider when investigating a facility are listed in Table 3–1, below.

Beginning a CRE exercise program

If your self-assessment leads you to try to improve your CRE, you will need an exercise program designed specifically to help you meet that goal. To succeed with the program, however, will mean applying the two basic principles of fitness training—specificity and progressive overload.

Specificity

The training principle of specificity can help you narrow your choice to the activities best suited for improvement of CRE. These are the ones that use large muscle groups steadily and rhythmically—activities such as walking, jogging, swimming, bicycling, cross-country skiing, rope skipping, and hiking. All of these are effective because they require large amounts of energy, thus burning a large number of calories. (This makes many of these same activities well suited for reducing body fat or losing weight.) Keeping track of the number of calories burned in a particular

---

*In an article on annual physicals published in the October 1980 issue of *Consumer Reports*, Consumers Union's medical consultants dismissed the usefulness of cardiac stress testing in a routine physical examination for people without symptoms of coronary heart disease or coronary heart disease risk factors as "an extravagant waste of money." What's more, *Consumer Reports* noted, stress tests may also fail to detect coronary heart disease in a small number of people who actually have it.

Table 3–1

Checklist for Selecting a Cardiac Stress Test Facility

Listed below are questions to help you select the best possible facility to administer a cardiac stress test. If there is a choice of facilities in your area, you may prefer the one whose staff gives the greatest number of affirmative responses. The first question, in the opinion of Consumers Union's medical consultants, is the most important.

	Yes	No
1. Is monitoring continued throughout the cool-down and recovery periods?		
2. Is the supervising physician a board-certified cardiologist, experienced in stress testing?		
3. Will a physician examine your cardiovascular system before the test?		
4. Will you be given a resting electrocardiogram before the test?		
5. Does the physician ask about any medication you may be using that might affect the electrocardiogram?		
6. Is a warm-up part of the test?		
7. Is an electrocardiogram administered while you are hyperventilating?		
8. Is a progressive multistage treadmill test utilized?		
9. Is intermittent on-going multilead monitoring of the electrocardiogram performed by the tester? (Beginning before and continuing until after testing is completed?)		
Is an oscilloscope used?		
Is a written recorder used?		
10. Will your blood pressure be monitored continuously during the test?		
11. Is the test continued until the maximum heart rate is achieved (unless electrocardiogram changes, or there are other symptoms, or fatigue occurs, or until the subject wishes to stop)?		
12. Is there an emergency plan: A defibrillator, drug kit, ready access to a hospital?		

exercise program is a convenient way to measure the energy requirement of the activity. The greater the amount of energy expended, the greater the amount of oxygen that your cardiorespiratory system will deliver to the muscles.

Activities effective for CRE are self-paced—you can control progressive overload by adjusting the intensity, duration, and frequency of your exercise sessions as your fitness increases. Such adjustments may be more difficult with competitive sports. If you choose tennis or basketball as your CRE exercise, for example, the intensity of your play may not be within your control. Your skills may be so minimal that you won't be active enough to get a training effect. Or you may get discouraged or bored if your level of skills is better or worse than those of the competition. Or in the excitement of the game, you may push yourself beyond a comfortable level of intensity.

Progressive overload

No matter which specific activity you choose, you will need to base your exercise program on the principle of progressive overload. The idea is to begin with your current exercise level and gradually expose your body to increasing demands. The way you achieve overload will depend on which combinations of intensity, duration, and frequency of workout suits you best. In a twenty-week study comparing walking and jogging, for example, one group of men participated in fast walking for forty minutes, four days a week while another group jogged for thirty minutes, three days a week. The higher intensity of the jogging program was offset by the increased duration and frequency of the walking program, so that both groups expended the same total amount of energy each week. The amount of overload—and the extent of CRE improvement—was the same in both groups.

So if you stick to proper combinations of intensity, duration, and frequency, you can improve CRE whether you walk, jog, swim, cycle, ski, skip rope, or hike. Even though these activities demand different levels of exertion, thus burning different numbers of calories per minute, all can produce CRE training effects. Choose the one that most appeals to you and that you can expect to practice regularly all year round. (Keep in mind that although jogging three miles in thirty minutes every other day may be sufficient if you wish to improve and maintain general cardiorespiratory fitness, such a regimen would not make you a competitive runner.)

Intensity

You won't get CRE training effects unless the intensity of your workout is high enough to raise your heart rate sufficiently above its usual resting level and to keep it there for at least fifteen minutes. You need not raise your heart rate to its maximum rate to get CRE improvement,

61

however. Just keep your heart rate higher than its resting rate and lower than its maximum rate—within what we call the exercise benefit zone (EBZ). Your maximum heart rate (MHR) and EBZ can both be established fairly simply by following the procedures outlined below.

MHR and EBZ. If you have had a cardiac stress test that took your heart rate to maximum, the test facility can probably tell you your precise maximum heart rate per minute—the heart rate you achieved at maximum intensity during the test period. Stress test data are not essential, however. You can estimate your maximum heart rate very easily by subtracting your age from the figure 220. If you are thirty years old, then, your estimated maximum heart rate is 190.

Finding your exercise benefit zone—between 70 and 85 percent of maximum heart rate—is almost as simple. All you have to do is make two calculations, based on the MHR, to establish your EBZ.* Once you have a maximum heart rate—either exact or estimated—just multiply it by .70 to find the lower threshold of your EBZ and by .85 to find the upper limit. Table 3–2 shows estimated MHRs and EBZs for the typical male and female for ages fifteen through seventy-five. For example, if you are fifty years old, your estimated MHR is 170 and your EBZ is between 119 and 145. To achieve CRE training effects when you exercise, you would need to maintain your heart rate within your EBZ for fifteen minutes or more per exercise session.

Remember, you need not exercise at maximum heart rate to achieve training effects. As long as you raise your heart rate into the EBZ, you will make progress. Within that range of intensity, you can vary the amount of your overload at will. The magnitude of training effects increases with the extent of the overload, but you can keep intensity relatively low and still get training effects by overloading duration or frequency.

All you must do to achieve improvement in CRE is to maintain your heart rate within your EBZ during your regular exercise sessions. It is not necessary to raise your heart rate to higher and higher levels. Just stay in your EBZ. For example, M.J., a fifty-two-year-old New Yorker, told Consumers Union that he regularly runs a seven-mile course with a heart rate of 130 beats per minute. When he established this routine, he was running the course in about seventy minutes. Some months later his time had dropped to sixty-seven minutes, and a month after that it was down to

---

*The American College of Sports Medicine recommends, and many people use, a procedure known as the Karvonen method to calculate the EBZ. The Karvonen method considers the EBZ as between 60 and 90 percent of *maximum heart rate reserve:* Maximum heart rate minus resting heart rate multiplied by .60 plus resting heart rate equals 60 percent of heart rate reserve. We prefer a simpler calculation that places the EBZ between 70 and 85 percent of MHR, with the resting heart rate not included in the computation.

Table 3-2

Estimated Maximum Heart Rate and Exercise Benefit Zone by Age

Subtract your age from 220 to get your estimated maximum heart rate (MHR). Find that figure on the top line of the Table. Below the figure you can find the upper threshold and the lower threshold of your EBZ. Example: If you are 50 years old, your estimated MHR is 170 (220−50) and your EBZ thresholds are 145 (upper) and 119 (lower).

Age in years	15	20	25	30	35	40	45	50	55	60	65	70	75
Estimated maximum heart rate (MHR) (beats per minute)	205	200	195	190	185	180	175	170	165	160	155	150	145
Upper threshold EBZ (85 percent level)	174	170	166	162	157	153	149	145	140	136	132	128	123
Lower threshold EBZ (70 percent level)	144	140	137	133	130	126	123	119	116	112	109	105	102

EXERCISE BENEFIT ZONE

sixty-five minutes. Both distance and heart rate remained the same but M.J.'s increase in CRE let him increase the speed of his run, thus shortening the duration of his exercise period.

Taking your pulse. To be sure that you are exercising hard enough to keep your heart rate within your EBZ, you may have to learn how to take your pulse.* You can do this using either the radial artery or the carotid artery; both are near enough to the skin for you to feel them easily. To locate the radial artery, place the tips of the middle three fingers of your right hand on the left wrist in the little groove below the base of your left thumb. To locate the carotid artery, place the tips of the three middle fingers of one hand on your neck under the jaw bone, about midway between the chin and the ear. (See illustration.) Hold your fingertips

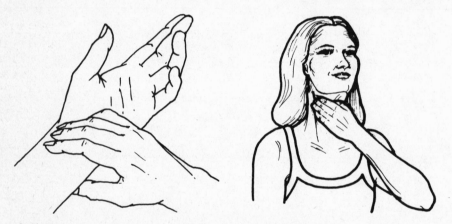

gently but firmly on one of these pressure points, and you will be able to feel the artery pulsating—each pulsation reflecting a heart beat. Using a stopwatch (push the start button and begin counting) or a watch with a sweep-second hand, count the number of pulse beats in ten seconds. To determine your heart rate per minute, multiply by 6.

---

*The January 1980 issue of *Consumer Reports* discussed a number of automated pulse recorders. These gadgets could help people under close medical supervision, but Consumers Union's medical consultants thought they were cumbersome and expensive. The February 1980 issue of *Consumer Reports* discussed a heart rate monitor that not only recorded your pulse but let you program the upper and lower heart rate limits that define your EBZ. An alarm sounded when your pulse was outside your EBZ. This equipment had its flaws (erratic readings, rather complex program sequences, and the like), and was expensive. But it might be worth the investment if your physician says your heart rate should be measured and controlled during exericse.

Table 3–3 can be used to identify your EBZ in terms of your ten-second pulse rate. That can save you the trouble of having to multiply in the midst of a workout. Start counting your pulse immediately after exercising because the heart rate drops significantly within fifteen seconds. By stopping your exercise briefly and taking your pulse right

---

Table 3–3

Determining Your Exercise Benefit Zone

To improve CRE, an exercise should bring your heart rate to your exercise benefit zone (EBZ)—between 70 and 85 percent of your maximum heart rate (MHR) —and should maintain your heart rate within your EBZ. The Table below provides estimated MHR per minute and the EBZ for various ages. (You can approximate your MHR by subtracting your age from 220.) To guide your pulse-taking during exercise, refer to the 10-second conversion for each set of MHR data below. The Table also gives you the number of beats per minute at the 70 percent and 85 percent level of EBZ.

Age	Estimated MHR per minute	Exercise benefit zone			
		70% estimated MHR		85% estimated MHR	
		60 sec.	10 sec.	60 sec.	10 sec.
15	205	144	24	174	29
20	200	140	23	170	28
25	195	137	23	166	28
30	190	133	22	162	27
35	185	130	22	157	26
40	180	126	21	153	26
45	175	123	21	149	25
50	170	119	20	145	24
55	165	116	19	140	24
60	160	112	19	136	23
65	155	109	18	132	22
70	150	105	18	128	21
75	145	102	17	123	21

away, you can readily determine whether your exercise is keeping your heart rate within your EBZ.

If you don't want to interrupt your exercise to take your pulse, try the "talk test": You are probably at the lower end of your EBZ if you can comfortably hold a conversation while exercising. With experience, some people can learn to judge whether they are in the EBZ without stopping to check their pulse.

The EBZ is, at best, an approximation. It is important for you to monitor how your body feels on any particular day. You may have to increase or reduce your exercise intensity to adapt to a variety of circumstances. Your reaction to exercise may vary in response to such environmental factors as temperature, humidity, or altitude, or to such personal variables as infection, medication, fatigue, and psychological stress.

Duration

The duration of an exercise period will depend, of course, on how strenuous the exercise is. In general, the harder you work, the shorter the time you must spend to achieve the desired effect. But if you are exercising at high intensity near the upper limit of your EBZ, you may exhaust yourself quickly. If you are exercising close to the lower threshold of your EBZ, you will be able to continue longer.

There is some evidence that you can get a training effect by working at or above the upper limit of your EBZ for as little as five or ten minutes. But because the potential for injury—especially among beginners—is greater with more strenuous exercise, the likelihood of continued improvement is lower. Our senior authors recommend, along with most authorities, that a CRE exercise period should last at least fifteen minutes (not including warm-up or cool-down). For an exerciser to sustain an activity for the minimum fifteen minutes may mean having to work at the lower end of the EBZ. Our senior authors' experience with thousands of York College students age eighteen to over seventy suggest that at the beginning of an exercise program your activity period should last fifteen minutes and that, as you become adjusted to the work load, you should add increased time at a rate of no more than 10 percent a week.

Beginners should progress very gradually to greater durations and higher intensities. Studies with joggers indicate that low-intensity exercise for long durations helps avoid injuries and minimize discomfort. At least eight or ten weeks of slowly increasing the duration of training may be necessary for most beginners. It may even be advisable to start at an intensity considerably below your EBZ until your muscles adjust to the demands of your program. As you increase the intensity of the workout, and as the training effects begin to accrue, you may find yourself increasing the duration of your exercise sessions simply because they have become an enjoyable experience.

N.L., a fifty-year-old woman from Scarsdale, New York, told Consumers Union that when she first took up running she could barely finish one-quarter of a mile. She found it boring and mindless, but persisted because she felt it was "doing her a lot of good." After a year of training, her endurance had increased until she could cover six miles regularly in sixty-three minutes. She slept "amazingly well" and could eat "practically anything without putting on weight." At that point, she bought her second pair of running shoes, joined a local running club, and admitted that somewhere between three miles and five miles, she had actually begun to enjoy it.

The higher the intensity or the longer the duration of the exercise session (or possibly both, as you get used to the activity), the greater will be the improvement in CRE. A little experimentation with the structure of your exercise regimen will help you find the best way to adjust intensity and duration to get maximum improvement in CRE. The combinations are almost infinite and can always be varied to suit your particular needs and interests.

Frequency

Frequency of exercise, for the beginner, need not be more than three or four days a week for most activities. In fact, jogging and running more frequently than that may increase the chance of injury, particularly for the beginner. Three days a week, or about every other day, is adequate to achieve improvement in CRE. (Athletes usually require more training time.)

Some people, however, don't like to skip a day between exercising. If you prefer a routine of, say, six days a week, feel rested enough before each workout, and have no muscular or joint problems (as is often reported by overzealous joggers), the almost daily routine may help to develop even higher levels of CRE. Such a schedule would certainly be useful if you also wanted to achieve and maintain lean body composition. If you want to exercise more than every other day, it might be wise to alternate the type of CRE exercise you do, especially if you are prone to injury and want to avoid muscular or joint problems. For example, you might run one day and swim the next or you might alternate bicycling one day with taking a brisk walk the next.

It's important to continue exercising. When you are inactive, deconditioning occurs fairly quickly. A study from the Universities of Maryland and Kentucky reported on a group of women who exercised for ten weeks and made significant gains in CRE. When they later dropped their training for five weeks, they lost almost 70 percent of their CRE gains. After ten weeks without exercise, they were back where they had started before the training program began. In another study, conducted by investigators at Wake Forest University, a group of men jogged eight miles a week for twenty weeks. Twelve weeks later, those who had dropped down to less than five miles a week had lost about 50 percent of their gains. Those who kept to a routine of about eight miles a week continued to improve in CRE.

These studies confirm our belief that a workout within the EBZ about every other day is necessary to maintain cardiorespiratory fitness. Less frequent exercise will not only fall short of producing training effects, it may also allow deconditioning to occur.

Calories as a measure of CRE exercise

The amount of work you do in the exercise regimen you select depends on how you adjust and combine intensity, duration, and frequency to achieve progressive overload. One measure of that work is the energy you expend in doing it. And the simplest way to keep track of energy is by noting the number of calories you burn. If the activity you choose meets the basic principles of specificity and progressive overload and if you know the total calories you burn in that activity, you can judge whether your exercise regimen is appropriate for achieving CRE training effects.

As discussed on page 73, the calorie is a unit of heat. It's commonly used to indicate not only the potential energy in food, but also the energy expended to perform work. (Table 4–1 on page 78 lists a broad range of activities that are more fully described in Chapters 7 and 8.) By adjusting intensity, duration, and frequency in various combinations, you can raise or lower the total number of calories you expend in your exercise sessions.

Table 3–4 illustrates how beginners with low CRE as well as the highly fit can use varied combinations of duration and frequency to achieve CRE goals.

The CRE potential of an activity depends on its ability to bring the heart rate into the EBZ. An activity that keeps your heart rate at the low end of the EBZ is a low-intensity activity. And one that raises your heart rate to the upper limits is a high-intensity activity.

If you choose an activity that burns more calories per minute than another activity—a high-intensity activity, for example, such as running instead of walking—you might be able to shorten the amount of time you need to spend on your exercise sessions to achieve your CRE goal. Or you could perform a high-intensity exercise at the top range of your EBZ: You could run at 85 percent of your maximum heart rate, which would burn more calories per minute than running at 70 percent.

But a high-intensity exercise won't necessarily improve CRE more than a low-intensity one (or exercising at the low end of your EBZ). In fact, exercise done at lower intensity may burn more calories overall, because it can usually be continued for longer periods at reduced intensity. For instance, pedaling your bike uphill is a high-intensity activity burning many more calories per minute than pedaling at the same speed on a level road. But you can keep up the low-intensity pedaling on the level road longer and thus burn more calories in a single session than in the brief but more intense uphill effort.

Some authorities believe a minimum number of calories must be expended if exercise is to provide protection against heart attack. A retrospective study by Ralph S. Paffenbarger, Jr., a professor of epidemiology at Stanford University, showed that Harvard alumni who burned 2,000 or more calories a week through exercise had fewer heart attacks than those who got less exercise. (Interestingly enough, Paffenbarger found that former varsity athletes who did not maintain a high level of activity after graduation were more at risk than those who had been nonathletes in their student days but who later became physically active.) Thomas Cureton, another authority on fitness, has suggested that burning 300 calories a session is helpful.

You may wish to undertake a CRE program using a calorie goal. If so, choose an exercise regimen that has the potential of relatively high caloric expenditure yet would permit you to reduce or increase intensity, duration, and frequency as your fitness level directs.

Table 3–4

Calorie Guide to CRE

The Table below shows how you can adjust duration and frequency when exercising within your EBZ (see pages 62–66) to establish the number of calories you need to burn per week to attain your CRE goals.

Calories used per week	Duration (minutes per session)	Frequency (days per week)	CRE level
250–500	15–20	3–4	Primarily for beginners with low CRE.
501–750	15–30	3–4	For those who wish to progress from low to moderate levels of CRE.
751–1,250	31–45	3–4	For those who wish to progress from moderate to high levels of CRE.
1,251–2,000	31–45	4–6	To achieve and maintain a very high level of CRE.
Over 2,000	31–60	4–6	To achieve and maintain a very high level of CRE; to try for possible cardiovascular benefits.

69

Exercise systems and CRE

You can make a good deal of progress on a well-planned CRE program suited to your interests and abilities. Your progress, however, can be affected by the exercise system you choose to follow. Many people who exercise for CRE use a *continuous rhythmic technique* (CRT), which involves jogging, cycling, or swimming at a set pace for a set time. This system has simplicity as its chief advantage: Once you calculate your EBZ, all you have to do is choose a pace that will maintain your heart rate within the EBZ for the duration of your workout. CRT involves a relatively slow pace, continued for long distances. As CRE improves, the pace gets picked up automatically. CRT practitioners seem to enjoy the system because its simplicity allows for a period of pure activity, a time when few decisions have to be made and the body can proceed "on automatic."

For beginners, CRT can have some disadvantages. Because of low CRE, they may become fatigued and fail to last through an exercise session. Or the simplicity of the format and the monotony of the pace may become boring, tempting them to give up.

One way to get around the negative effects of a program based on CRT is to interrupt the exercise with *interval training*. This system shortens the periods of high-intensity activity by introducing brief periods of rest or low-intensity activity. Interval training allows your body to recuperate partially from the high-intensity work, permitting you to complete a longer total period of work without becoming exhausted or bored. These intervals of high- and low-intensity activity can be repeated until you have finished the number of sets you planned to do.

Here's how interval training works. Suppose twenty minutes is your best time for jogging two miles while maintaining your heart rate within your EBZ. And suppose your rate of speed is six miles per hour (ten minutes per mile). With interval training, you can run one-half mile in five minutes (or even slightly faster), followed by a one-eighth-mile walk at three miles per hour. If you alternate these four times, your total distance will be two and one-half miles. The exercise duration will then become thirty minutes instead of the twenty minutes that was your manageable limit with continuous rhythmic activity. And you will have burned approximately 280 calories instead of 250.

4

Body Composition

"In my lifetime I suppose I have lost approximately 500 pounds!" So began a letter from H.H., a forty-five-year-old woman from Felton, Delaware. Like many other *Consumer Reports* readers, she undertook a physical fitness program primarily to lose weight.

Others told Consumers Union they wanted to firm up or slim down. For many, the decision to lose weight or to shed fat had a tone of determination. "Ten years ago at age thirty-two," reported M.P. of Lorain, Ohio, describing his moment of truth, "I stood nude before a full-length mirror and, frowning with disgust, realized that my chest had slid down into my belly." He still weighed the same 200 pounds he had as a seventeen-year-old football player, but his waist was now 40 inches. L.R., a twenty-six-year-old woman from Hollywood, California, had a similar confrontation. "I finally couldn't pretend any more," she confessed to Consumers Union. "When I looked in the mirror, I could see it. . . . I decided it had to stop there."

For some people, the turning point came in the physician's office. D.N., a sixty-six-year-old artist from St. Louis, discovered some years ago that he had a tendency toward diabetes. Following his doctor's advice, he took off fifteen pounds with the aid of a stationary bicycle and calisthenics. "Thanks to the loss of weight and the increase in the amount of exercise," wrote D.N., "I have been able to control my blood sugar without drugs." Ironically, D.N. had begun his forty-year commitment to exercise when he joined a "Y" to *gain* weight. After five years, he had progressed from 127 to 165 pounds, and then worked to keep himself at that weight by exercising at least three times a week.

Most people, of course, want to *lose* weight. R.M., at age fifty-nine, said she was surprised to learn at her annual physical that she had gained eight pounds in the past year. The South Bend, Indiana, woman, at 5 foot 7 inches tall and 137 pounds, was not fat, but her doctor reminded her that if she gained another eight pounds the next year she would probably be heavier than she'd like. In about sixteen months of diet and exercise, she got her weight down to 120 pounds.

Overweight, overfat, and obese

It's no surprise that physicians often figure so prominently in reports of weight loss. Although obesity is not a primary risk factor for coronary heart disease, it can be a danger signal, particularly in someone with one or more of the known risk factors (see page 20). Loss of weight, especially when it's the side effect of a regular exercise program, may lessen the chance of coronary heart disease, speed rehabilitation after heart attack, and prevent a recurrence. Problems related to diabetes, gallbladder disease, and hypertension (high blood pressure) may also be reduced by weight loss.

Estimates vary, but there are probably 50 to 80 million Americans—up to half the adult and adolescent population—who are overweight. What this means in most cases is that these people weigh more than the so-called ideal weight for their height and build. Others may not be overweight by the charts but they feel—and look—overfat. In contrast, the charts may lump a few into the overweight category when their excess weight is actually due to muscle development rather than too much body fat.

If you've done any of the self-assessment tests in Chapter 1 to determine the proportion of body fat to muscle, you should know how you rate in terms of body composition. For men, more than 25 percent body fat indicates obesity; men whose body fat is between 20 and 25 percent are overfat. Women with more than 35 percent body fat are considered to be obese; with more than 30 percent, they are overfat.

The nature of obesity (and overfatness) can be mystifying. Not until the 1960s was there a breakthrough in understanding obesity. It was then that Jules Hirsch and his colleagues at Rockefeller University in New York City showed that fat people have extra-large fat cells and, interestingly, that they have more fat cells than thinner people. When a fat person loses weight on a low-calorie diet, it is the size of each fat cell that decreases, not the number of fat cells. The number of fat cells probably remains constant from about adolescence onward.

Because of the significance of the childhood years in the development of fat cells, people concerned about children's health should—after consultation with a physician—encourage calorie restriction when appropriate. And they should encourage regular, vigorous exercise for children. Obesity can never be cured. It can be controlled, however, by maintaining a balance between eating (the amount of calories ingested) and physical activity (the amount of calories burned). If young children and teenagers are encouraged to shun excess calories and to exercise regularly, the problem of obesity in their adulthood may be minimized.

72

If you were unable to assess your body composition by using any of the methods described in Chapter 1, you may be able to make a rough judgment on the basis of more casual evidence. Has your weight gone up continually over the years since you graduated from high school or college? If so, the additional weight has probably been in the form of fat. You may be a victim of "creeping obesity," like B.R., a thirty-six-year-old *Consumer Reports* reader from Spring, Texas, whose weight went from 136 to 180 in his first year at a desk job, or like M.S., thirty, who gained about twenty-five pounds in the nine years he worked in an office in Orlando, Florida.

As M.S. did, you may have been putting on weight slowly but steadily over a period of years. Even if you haven't gained an ounce since your early twenties, your activity level may have declined. If so, it is likely that some muscles may have decreased in size and some fat deposits may have increased in size. This process is inevitable with aging, but it proceeds at a slower rate in people who are physically active. As a result, you may decide that your goal is not so much weight reduction as fat reduction, or what many people call toning up the body—increasing muscular fitness and making muscles stronger.

Calories and energy

Whether your goal is to improve body composition or to reduce total weight, your approach will be the same: to lose fat. Almost always, steps taken to reduce body fat will also lower body weight. Theories and methods of weight control come and go, but most authorities now agree that weight control is best achieved by a combination of strategies calling for both a balanced diet and regular exercise. The positive effects on weight reduction of reduced dietary intake and increased exercise output are most readily illustrated in terms of calories.

A unit of measurement, a calorie (technically, a kilocalorie) is actually the amount of heat required to raise the temperature of one gram of water 1 degree (from 14.5 to 15.5 degrees centigrade). Calories are used to measure the potential energy value of the food people eat and of the energy people expend in performing work.

One pound of body fat is equal to roughly 3,500 calories. If the food you eat in a day supplies 3,500 calories and you burn 3,500 calories in doing the day's work, you are in *neutral calorie balance:* You will neither gain nor lose weight. If, however, the next day you have a lighter work schedule, and if you take in 4,000 calories and you burn only 2,300 calories, you will have a *positive calorie balance* of 1,700 calories. These 1,700 surplus calories—whether consumed as protein, carbohydrate, or fat—will show up eventually as about one-half pound of body fat, stored in fat cells, ready to be converted into a reserve supply of energy should the need arise. If no need arises, the fat deposits remain where they are.

If on the following day you resume your normal work load, expending 3,500 calories but taking in only 1,800 calories, you will be in *negative calorie balance* to the tune of 1,700 calories. Your body will have to call upon its reserve of fat for your energy needs that day. Theoretically, you would lose about one-half pound of fat. If you stay in positive calorie balance for a significant time by either eating more or exercising less, you will gain weight by adding fat to your body. If you stay in negative calorie balance for a prolonged period by either eating less or exercising more, you will lose weight by using up some of your fat reserve. If you stay in neutral calorie balance, using up all the calories you take in each day, your weight will not change. Theoretically, it's as simple as that.

As most of us know, however, it isn't that simple at all. Even a small regular increase in daily calorie intake can markedly affect your weight. Suppose you begin to consume 250 extra calories a day—say, two thick slices of bread and butter—without any change in your activity pattern. You could then count on gaining about a pound every two weeks. At the end of a year, you would have put on some twenty-six pounds—just from a mere 250 more calories a day. It would be a different story, of course, if you began a new exercise program or increased your activities when you increased your food intake. That way you could maintain a neutral calorie balance or even work for a negative calorie balance—and lose weight.

Crash diets

Resist the temptation to begin your weight reduction campaign by going on a crash diet. Most of these so-called miracle cures for obesity require such drastic changes in your regular eating habits that you're not likely to stick with them for very long. And if you do maintain the diet, you could be compromising your health. Instead, we suggest you take a more conservative approach to weight loss. It requires more perseverance but offers a greater probability of success because it calls for less disruption of your customary eating patterns.

Most crash diets are based on ill-considered, half-understood, or pseudoscientific theories. Some of these diets place a potentially dangerous emphasis on certain kinds of foods to the neglect or exclusion of others. Many fad diets rely on a drastic reduction in or even elimination of dietary carbohydrate. Cutting back on carbohydrate reduces the glycogen (stored carbohydrate) in muscles and liver. With every gram of lost carbohydrate there is also a loss of about three grams of body water. The dramatic loss of five or more pounds almost immediately after you go on such a diet is almost entirely attributable to a sudden increase in urinary output. You have not lost any fat—just fluid. Fat cannot usually be lost that rapidly. And weight loss due to fluid loss is easily regained. What seemed like instant success could turn into a discouraging setback.

Moreover, if you increase your activity level to create a negative calorie balance, you will need a well-balanced diet. It would be imprudent, if not downright dangerous, to undertake an exercise program without meeting your nutritional needs. It would be much wiser to reduce your caloric intake slightly, being sure to include adequate protein, carbohydrate, fat, vitamins, and minerals. At the same time, increase your activity enough to ensure a negative calorie balance. With such a regimen, you should be able to lose weight slowly but steadily.

Exercise and diet

One of our senior authors used to ask the prospective physical education teachers in his classes whether they thought exercise had any part in weight reduction. The majority—at the beginning of the term, at any rate—ruled out exercise, insisting that only diet was important. They claimed it was impossible—or at least impracticable—to lose weight through exercise. You would have to jog seven hours to burn the 3,500 calories needed to lose one pound, their argument went. Who could jog for seven hours? The fallacy, of course, is that you need not burn all 3,500 calories at one time, any more than you would necessarily take in the 3,500 calories all at one meal. Actually, if you jog only a half-hour a day, after fourteen days you will have completed seven hours of jogging. At the rate of 500 calories an hour, you would have established a negative calorie balance of 3,500 calories over those two weeks—provided, of course, that you maintained your normal calorie intake and carried on all your other activities as usual during those two weeks.

Losing one pound in two weeks may not seem like much, especially contrasted with the lure of a crash diet that promises a twenty-pound loss in the same time. But if you were to maintain prudent eating patterns and jog every day for a year, you would actually lose twenty-six pounds, six more than the crash diet tempted you with. And you would have a much better chance of keeping the weight off than if you had starved yourself for two weeks on a crash diet. If, in addition to jogging, you also decreased your caloric intake by as little as 250 calories a day (cutting out those two thick slices of bread and butter, for example), you would create an even greater negative calorie balance, and thus lose weight a bit more rapidly than by exercise alone.

Appetite and exercise

People used to think that appetite invariably increases with exercise. That is usually not the case, especially with part-time exercisers who work out three to five days a week for a relatively brief time. Studies have shown that, over a period of months, most people who exercise strenuously for more than thirty minutes but less than one hour experience little if any change in appetite and they succeed in losing weight.

An unusually heavy work load, however, does affect appetite. A construction worker who does six to seven hours of heavy muscular labor

75

day in and day out or a dancer who spends six to seven hours a day in class, rehearsal, and performance may require diets relatively high in calories to support their extremely high levels of activity. Similarly, the average person who spends a long vacation day on a ski trail or backpacking—and burns unaccustomed amounts of calories—will probably be ravenous at dinner. But this increase in appetite does not hold true for people who exercise regularly for shorter time spans. And even those who do get an increase in appetite—and therefore increase their food intake some-what—still manage to lose weight as long as they are careful to remain in negative calorie balance.

Diet without exercise

If you want to improve your body composition as well as lose weight —that is, if your self-assessment has shown that you're not merely over-weight but overfat—you probably want to increase your ratio of muscle to fat while you take off excess pounds. There is some evidence that dieting alone may cause you to lose muscle as well as fat. In one controlled study, for example, a group of twenty-five overweight women lost between 10.6 and 12 pounds in sixteen weeks. One subgroup of the women reduced their daily food intake by 500 calories. Another subgroup increased their daily activities to burn an additional 500 calories each. The remainder reduced their dietary intake by just 250 calories—maintaining the same percentage relationship among protein, carbohydrate, and fat—and stepped up their exercise to burn 250 additional calories. All three groups lost roughly the same amount of weight. But the diet-only group lost lean muscle tissue as well as body fat, while the exercise-only group and the diet-and-exercise group both gained in muscle rather than lost. What's more, they lost more fat than did the diet-only group.

Choosing a sensible regimen

A reasonable goal for weight loss is no more than one pound a week. Over a year's time, even if you lost one-half pound a week, you'd be lighter by about twenty-six pounds. To lessen the chance of losing lean muscle tissue along with fat, you should increase your level of exercise as well as decrease calorie intake while accomplishing the weight loss.

Particularly important for changing body composition and for losing weight are the duration and frequency of your exercise program. (Inten-sity is less important for improvement in this fitness component.) For most people, a duration of thirty minutes and a frequency of at least three times a week seem to be the *minimum* requirements for altering body composition and achieving weight loss.

In one study, for example, women who were 10 to 60 percent over-weight did not begin to lose weight until the duration of a walking program was more than thirty minutes a day. Over a year, the women—

who were subject to no dietary restrictions—lost an average of twenty-two pounds each. In another study, thirty-minute sessions twice a week of a walking/jogging/running program were not enough to change body composition, while the same program four times a week did reduce body fat significantly.

Increasing duration and frequency can increase the rate of change. Consider R.G., who described for Consumers Union his regimen of running about six miles in forty-five minutes almost every day. "When I started running," he wrote, "I was twenty-eight years old, 160 pounds, 5 feet 9 inches. I knew that I burned 100 calories for every mile that I ran, so I expected to lose some weight. But I did not expect to now weigh about 135 pounds, a loss of twenty-five pounds!" R.G. says he hadn't wanted to lose that much weight, and even had increased his food intake by snacking. He now feels "fantastic at 135 pounds."

Which exercise is best?

Cardiorespiratory endurance (CRE)—or aerobic—activities, such as walking, jogging, running, swimming, and bicycling, are the most useful for losing weight because they eventually burn more calories than do muscle-strengthening exercises, such as weight training or calisthenics. Weight training, however, can increase muscle tissue and thereby increase the proportion of muscle to fat. The sedentary and relatively inactive person may take comfort in the knowledge that walking is as effective for weight loss as bicycling or running, as long as you pay proper attention to duration and frequency of exercise. The overweight women in the walking program cited earlier walked for more than thirty minutes a day every day for a year and—with no dietary restrictions at all—lost from ten to thirty-eight pounds.

Remember that you can increase the total calories expended while performing an activity if you prolong duration even if you have to reduce intensity to do so. In other words, to change body composition you probably would be better off walking for an hour than jogging for twenty minutes. Calories do count, after all, but they count much more if you count them on the road as well as on the plate.

To decide which exercise to select as part of a body composition regimen, consult Table 4–1, which lists a variety of fitness activities and the calories expended for each. (These activities are a sampling of those listed in Chapter 8.)

A strategy for changing body composition need not be based exclusively on a formal exercise program, however. Practically any everyday activity uses up calories. Several *Consumer Reports* readers told us they had healthy appetites but maintained their weight by combining regular exercise with a vigorous approach to routine daily tasks. For example, M.G., a twenty-four-year-old secretary from New York who took a daily jog down Fifth Avenue on her lunch hour, wrote that she looks on almost everything she does as potential exercise: "Even when I do housework I try to do it in a brisk manner and not just clean." A seventy-year-old retired man declares himself in excellent health although he exercises only occasionally. He explained, "I think good steady activity around the house takes the place of sporadic exercise."

Table 4–2 lists a sampling of nonsport activities and their calorie

Table 4–1

Estimated Calorie Costs of Fitness Activities

This Table lists calorie costs for a sampling of the fitness activities included in Chapter 8. The second column shows estimated costs of calories per minute per pound of body weight. Multiply your body weight by the figure in the second column to get your estimated calorie cost per minute for an exercise or activity.

Activity	Cal./min./lb.
Aerobic dance (vigorous)	.062
Basketball (vigorous, full court)	.097
Bicycling (13 mph)	.071
Canoeing (flat water, 4 mph)	.045
Cross-country skiing (8 mph)	.104
Golf (twosome carrying clubs)	.045
Handball (skilled, singles)	.078
Horseback riding (trot)	.052
Jogging (5 mph)	.060
Rowing (vigorous)	.097
Running (8 mph)	.104
Snowshoeing (2.5 mph)	.060
Soccer (vigorous)	.097
Swimming (55 yds./min.)	.088
Table tennis (skilled)	.045
Tennis (beginner)	.032
Walking (4.5 mph)	.048

Table 4–2

Estimated Calorie Costs of Nonsport Activities

This Table lists calorie costs for a sampling of nonsport activities. The second column shows estimated costs of calories per minute per pound of body weight. Multiply your body weight by the figure in the second column to get your estimated calorie cost per minute for an activity.

Activity	Cal./min./lb.
Bathing, dressing, undressing	.021
Bed-making (and stripping)	.031
Chopping wood	.049
Cleaning windows	.024
Driving a car	.020
Eating while seated	.011
Gardening: Digging	.062
Hedging	.034
Raking	.024
Weeding	.038
Ironing	.029
Kneading dough	.023
Laundry (taking out and hanging)	.027
Mopping floors	.024
Painting house (outside)	.034
Peeling potatoes	.019
Piano playing	.018
Plastering walls	.023
Sawing wood (crosscut saw)	.058
Shining shoes	.017
Shoveling snow	.052
Writing while seated	.013

costs. To determine the value of these nonsport activities for weight reduction, apply the same criteria as you would for any of the exercises or activities listed in Table 4–1. Obviously, if you're going to rely on dressing, eating your meals, and writing letters to help you lose weight, you won't make much progress. Such activities use few calories per minute and don't usually last for long. However, if you weed a garden regularly, paint your house, shovel snow, or even hang the wash, you're much more likely to experience weight loss. Such activities are more effective for weight loss than, say, getting dressed, because they expend more calories and require more of your time to do them. In fact, you're apt to burn calories at about the same rate as for many active sports. For even greater success in weight loss, supplement your exercise program—and your routine household chores—by eating a little less.

Can exercise reduce fat in particular parts of the body? No. Most authorities reject the concept of "spot reduction." Stored fat belongs to the whole body, not just to the area where it happens to be stored. When you exercise, fat is mobilized from *all* the fat cells of the body. Spot exercising may build muscle in a specific area and thus may firm it up. But there is no evidence that the fat itself will disappear.

CRE exercise is best for losing weight. It uses more and larger muscle groups, and thus burns more calories, than brief localized exercise of individual parts of the body. Again, losing weight is a matter of patience and perseverance. A nutritionally sound diet together with a CRE program designed to achieve a negative calorie balance will help you lose weight, and you're sure—eventually—to lose some fat on your hips or around your waist.

Will a rubber exercise suit, vibrating machine, massage, or sauna help you lose weight? A rubber exercise suit is useless for weight reduction, despite claims that it will help you sweat off fat. And after you've had a glass or two of fluid, even the loss of the fluid would not be sustained. In fact, dressing too warmly for exercise—which would include wearing a rubber suit—could even harm you as a result of dehydration.

Vibrators, massage, and saunas are just as ineffective for weight loss as rubber suits. An effective weight control program, as you know, requires activities that expend calories.

Advocates of the rubber suit and the sauna for weight loss also forget (or overlook) the fact that the body burns more calories when it's cool. If you exercise in a cool environment you would burn calories, which are units of heat, just to maintain your body temperature at 98.6°F. Therefore, the cooler the environment when you exercise, the more calories you're likely to expend.

Does weight training contribute to weight loss? Because weight training is an excellent exercise for muscle development, it will increase the percentage of muscle in your body composition at the expense of the fat. To lose weight, use weight training to supplement an activity high in caloric expenditure, such as walking, jogging, running, swimming, or bicycling. These activities, which can be sustained over a long duration, burn many calories; if repeated regularly, they should help you lose weight. Combined with weight training, they give you a balanced program leading to a loss of fat and an increase in muscle.

Can exercise and diet help you gain weight? By applying the same principle of calorie balance that works for weight reduction, you can also adjust your calorie intake to exceed your energy expenditure. Just as a negative calorie balance will cause you to lose weight, so a positive calorie balance will cause you to gain. Increase your dietary intake by 500 calories each day, and you should be able to gain one pound in two weeks. If your activity level goes up, you can eat more—and be sure that you eat enough so that you don't burn more calories than you take in.

Because most people prefer to put on lean, muscular weight rather than flab or fat, and because muscle is more dense than fat, you should try to increase your body's total muscle mass. Begin by following the basic weight training model program in Chapter 7, but use fewer repetitions for each exercise. By doing only 6 to 10 repetitions, you will stimulate muscle growth without burning too many calories. If you're also interested in increasing your CRE, be careful to do no more than the minimum requirements for a CRE program. And, once again, be sure that you do not burn more calories than you take in.

What happens to your muscles if you give up exercise? Once you become inactive, the process of deconditioning begins: Muscle tissue is gradually lost. And fat is added if you continue to eat at the same levels as when you were physically active. Because one pound of fat is about five times the mass of one pound of muscle, you'll probably notice a change in body composition even if you're able to maintain your weight.

Is it safe for an obese and sedentary person to begin an exercise program for weight reduction? Yes, subject to the medical guidelines in Chapter 1. Getting started slowly is important for anyone who begins a new conditioning program. In this case, it would be crucial to use a program designed to begin with a very low overload. You may lose no weight at all for the first few weeks because muscles and the cardiorespiratory system will need some time to adjust to the new loads. You must be able to sustain a high enough level of activity for a long enough time before you can begin to burn those extra calories and shed fat. Patience is the most important element when you begin this kind of program. After the first few weeks, you should make significant and steady progress.

81

As we warned earlier in the chapter, resist the lure of crash diets. Weight loss on a crash diet is actually loss of fluid in most cases. It can be rapid but almost inevitably will not be maintained. A more gradual approach to weight loss—aiming for a maximum of one pound a week—will increase your chance of a permanent weight loss.

Can you do anything else besides diet and exercise to change body composition? Yes, a formal exercise program is not the only way you can increase your expenditure of energy. You can burn extra calories by avoiding many conveniences that make life unnecessarily easy. Take the stairs instead of the elevator if you have only a few flights to climb. Park your car two or three blocks from your destination. Better still, leave your car at home and bike or walk as much as possible. Walk briskly instead of strolling. In short, survey your home, your workplace, and your habits. Perhaps there are ways in which you can go a little farther and work a little harder if you forgo some step-saving and labor-saving "improvements." Altering your life-style in such seemingly insignificant ways can make a considerable difference—not only in weight control but in body composition and CRE as well—if you do it consistently over a long period of time.

5

Muscular Strength, Muscular Endurance, and Flexibility

If you're like most people, you probably pay little attention to the condition of your muscles, tendons, ligaments, and joints. During a typical day, you make demands on your body that it can meet quite comfortably. Only when the demand is unusual, or when an injury occurs, are you likely to become aware of the strength, endurance, and flexibility of your musculoskeletal system. Your car's power steering conks out, and you struggle to turn the wheel. Or you write thirty thank-you notes after a birthday party and you're left with writer's cramp. Or after climbing fifteen flights of stairs during a power failure, your muscles become so sore that the next day you can hardly walk across the room. Worse still, a serious illness or accident leaves you so weak that you can't sit up or even turn over in bed. All these examples of physical unfitness are caused, in large part, by poor performance in the components known as muscular strength, muscular endurance, and flexibility.

Muscular strength and endurance

If you have difficulty turning the lid of an ordinary jar, opening a window that's stuck, or lifting a heavy suitcase onto a closet shelf, it's probably the result of inadequate muscular strength. In Chapter 1 we defined muscular strength as the ability to exert maximum force, usually in a single exertion (as when you lift a heavy weight). But muscular strength can have less clear-cut applications. Weak abdominal muscles, for example, may contribute to low-back pain, just as weak thigh muscles may increase the chances of injuring your knee. And you need muscular strength to support the weight of your body against the pull of gravity. Even when you sit in a chair, your muscles are exerting force on various parts of your skeleton without your consciously thinking about it. When muscular strength falls below minimal levels, you may even begin to experience difficulty getting up from a chair, climbing one or two steps, or performing the lightest of your routine household tasks.

In general, your muscular strength is considered adequate if it lets you do all your daily routine comfortably. Muscular strength is not usually an end in itself, but a way to achieve success and satisfaction from whatever physical activities you choose. (For those interested in competitive sports, of course, muscular strength is essential.)

Muscular endurance is the ability to repeat a muscle contraction against resistance over and over again, or to hold a particular muscle in a contracted position for an extended time. Obviously, muscular endurance depends to some extent on muscular strength. Your muscles cannot repeat an action if they're too weak to perform it in the first place. Your muscular endurance also depends to some extent on your level of cardio-respiratory endurance (CRE). You cannot repeat an action many times over if your CRE cannot support the prolonged effort.

All body movements, including how you sit or stand, are brought about by the force of muscles pulling on tendons attached to bones. At every joint, opposing pairs of muscles coordinate to either flex or extend the joint. Some contract while others relax to bring about motion or to maintain position. In walking, for example, one group of muscles on the front of the thigh (the hip flexors) pulls the thigh bone forward while a group on the back of the thigh (the hip extensors) relaxes to permit the thigh to move forward. For the next step, the flexors relax and the extensors contract so the one leg moves rearward as the other leg steps forward. And so on, as you walk. It's the central nervous system that coordinates the muscles by orchestrating the contractions and relaxations at the precise moment to ensure that movements are made smoothly.

Each muscle is composed of numerous individual *muscle fibers,* which are grouped in *motor units* consisting of all the muscle fibers supplied by a single nerve. The number of muscle fibers in a motor unit may vary from as few as five and up to fifty in muscles used for sewing to as many as a thousand in muscles used for running. In each motor unit, the contraction of muscle fibers is triggered by an impulse from a nerve connected to the spinal cord and the higher centers of the central nervous system. When the muscle fibers in a motor unit contract, the force exerted by the motor unit is always the same: All the muscle fibers in the motor unit contract and they contract maximally (they are incapable of partial contractions). The force exerted by the whole muscle, however, varies with the number of motor units called into action. If you lift fifty pounds, for instance, you use fewer motor units than if you lift one hundred pounds.

How many muscle fibers you have does not change over your lifetime. But the individual muscle fibers can change in size, depending on how you use your muscles. The more you use a particular muscle, the larger and stronger its individual muscle fibers become, especially with resistance exercise such as weight training. An increase in muscle size is called muscle *hypertrophy*. A decrease in muscle size, muscle *atrophy*, occurs if muscle fibers are not used enough or if the nerve supplying them is injured. The body does not maintain a muscle or nerve if you no longer use it or if it becomes immobilized.

A case in point is the experience of a young Air Force sergeant who had been run over by a truck. Seriously injured, he had to remain in a full body cast for about six months—a very long period to be inactive. By the time his cast was removed and he came under the care of one of our senior authors (who was in charge of a physical reconditioning facility), the sergeant had lost more than 120 pounds. Formerly a basketball player on an Air Force team, he found he couldn't even raise his arms. He looked more like a concentration camp inmate than a patient who had been medically cared for in a hospital. His was a classic case of muscle atrophy due to prolonged inactivity.

The early stages of the sergeant's reconditioning consisted of passive exercise: Therapists helped him raise his arms and legs. Within a few days he could raise his own arms and even feed himself. A week later, he was using light weights to exercise his upper extremities while lying in bed. Gradually, he became able to do partial sit-ups. After two weeks, he was wheeled each day to the gymnasium where he progressed to exercises in a wheelchair or on a bench. He continued to improve with a reconditioning program based on weight training. As he became able to lift heavier and heavier weights, his body weight began to increase. Fitted with a leg brace, he learned how to walk with crutches. By his third month of recovery he had gained fifty pounds—and he reported that his upper body had become stronger than it had ever been.

To the sergeant the improvement appeared almost miraculous, but to the rehabilitation staff it was not very remarkable. By repeatedly using his muscles, the sergeant was causing individual muscle fibers to become larger and stronger. By progressively making greater and greater demands on specific muscle groups, he was gradually increasing muscular strength. His muscles increased in size and weight; his body weight increased; and he improved in all aspects of fitness. The sergeant's successful rehabilitation program had made use of the two basic training principles: specificity—selection of appropriate activities to achieve selected fitness goals; and progressive overload—increasing the work by gradually adding to the intensity, duration, and frequency of the exercise program.

Isotonics, isometrics, and isokinetics

You can improve your muscular strength and endurance with an exercise program using any one of three types of muscular contractions. The first occurs in any activity in which there is movement. For example, lifting a weight, as the sergeant did, involves *isotonic* muscular contractions. To lift a weight, you contract your bicep muscle, causing your elbow to bend; your forearm moves, and you lift the weight in your hand.

The second type of contraction takes place when a muscle contracts without shortening and therefore without movement. Any exercise against an immovable resistance is known as *isometric* exercise. If you place your palms against a wall and push as hard as you can, keeping your elbows bent, your muscles contract but without causing movement in the joint or limb. With isometrics, gains in muscular strength are limited, occurring only at the point of contraction. Weight training, as a form of isotonic exercise, has been compared with isometrics. Although both methods contribute to strength development, weight training has the advantage of producing strength throughout the full range of movement. This also maintains flexibility. Isometric exercise, however, can develop muscular strength in a limb that is in a cast where range of movement is limited.

A third type of contraction is called *isokinetic*. Here movement takes place as in an isotonic contraction. But unlike isotonics, where the resistance remains fixed (as with the weight you lift), during an isokinetic contraction the resistance adjusts itself to conform to the differences in muscular strength that exist at various points through the range of motion.

Prospects are promising for isokinetic exercise. One of its advantages in fitness training is that the speed of movement during the exercise can be made to simulate speeds specific to various sports. What's more, there appears to be little or no muscle soreness resulting from isokinetic exercise. For most people, however, isokinetic exercise is not yet readily available. (Some people can approximate isokinetic exercise by working with a partner who applies and adjusts manual resistance through the range of movement. Such approximations, however, are rarely as effective as isotonic exercises.)

Weight training

If your primary fitness goal is to improve muscular strength and endurance, a weight training program should give you the benefits you seek, along with improvements in flexibility and body composition as well. Even CRE benefits can be worked on during weight training if you use light weights and many repeat lifts (repetitions) to increase duration. (See, for example, the interval circuit training model program in Chapter 7.)

Weight training is exercise using barbells and dumbbells or machines offering comparable resistance, with weights and repetitions increased according to a specific overload system. The program is often referred to as progressive weight training (see Chapter 7 for a description of a model program). The equipment for weight training—barbells or dumbbells or both—is readily available and moderate in cost. For those who can afford it, more elaborate equipment is usually available at some fitness centers.

One caution before you begin a program of weight training. Because blood circulation tends to be impeded during weight training (and isometrics), such a program should not be undertaken without close medical supervision by people who have coronary heart disease, circulatory problems, or hypertension (high blood pressure). Consumers Union's medical consultants suggest that people who have any risk factors associated with coronary heart disease (see page 20) also check with their physician before undertaking a program in weight training (or isometrics).

By adjusting the amount of weight lifted and the number of repetitions, weight training can be adapted to emphasize either muscular strength or endurance. Heavy resistance with few repetitions works best for development of muscular strength. Light resistance with many repetitions is the key to muscular endurance.

An effective weight training program can be designed to supplement a general fitness program, one that includes CRE training and flexibility workouts as well. Because it's important to start any new exercise program cautiously, begin weight training with light resistance for just a few repetitions until you've mastered the exercise. Increase your work load gradually over the weeks. Despite such precautions, your muscles may feel sore after a workout. You can obtain some relief by gently stretching the affected muscle. As with any exercise, of course, it's essential to warm up and cool down (see stretching model program in Chapter 7).

Studies show that when you use a weight that can be lifted at maximum effort, about 6 to 8 repetitions are effective for increasing muscular strength. With that regimen, once you're able to perform 8 repetitions, add to the resistance by switching to a heavier weight and return to 6 repetitions. To improve muscular endurance, about 15 to 25 repetitions appear to be beneficial. And once you handle 25 repetitions in a muscular endurance program, switch to a heavier weight to increase resistance and begin once again at 15 repetitions. To be equally balanced for muscular strength and muscular endurance, use a system of 8 to 15 repetitions, with as much weight as you can handle. After you have achieved 15 repetitions, increase the weight and start with 8 repetitions. For best results, do 3 sets of repetitions every other day.

A basic program in weight training can be adapted to meet special needs and individual goals. You may want to design a weight training program to improve your performance in a particular sport. For example, if golf is your game, you would want to build muscular strength in your wrists and forearms as well as in the trunk muscles. Because golf does not require much muscular endurance, you would need to do only 6 or 8 repetitions of the weight training exercise you select. Swimmers would work for muscular strength and for endurance of the muscles of the chest, shoulders, upper back, and thighs. For most swimmers, 8 to 15 repetitions of a weight training exercise would be appropriate.

What does weight training accomplish? Most people use weight training to develop muscular strength and endurance as well as to improve muscle tone and physical appearance. Many also use weight training as a means of strengthening muscles and joints to minimize the chance of injury in competitive sports. Others use it to overcome an orthopedic problem, to prevent recurrence of one, or as part of an overall fitness and weight control program.

How does weight training differ from weight lifting? A competitive sport, *weight lifting* is an event in which the person lifting the greatest amount of weight wins. Weight lifters compete against each other according to body weight classifications, as boxers do. Each weight lifter gets three attempts at each of the two lifts that make up the competition. In the two-hand snatch, the athlete brings the weight up from the floor in one quick movement to a straight-arm overhead position. In the clean-and-jerk, which permits the use of heavier weights, the weight is first brought to the chest and then lifted overhead. The score is the sum of the greatest weight lifted in each of the two lifts.

Weight training is not a competitive sport. True, some weight trainers are also interested in competitive *body building*, which emphasizes the development of large well-defined muscles. Competitive body builders, sometimes called "iron pumpers," however, strive for a degree of muscular hypertrophy far beyond what most noncompetitive weight trainers regard as desirable.

Can women undertake weight training? Certainly. Women can respond as effectively to weight training as men to increase their general muscular strength and endurance and to prepare specific muscles for sports or other activities. In one supervised exercise program, untrained women, after a ten-week weight training program, were able to achieve greater increases in strength than the untrained men in the program.

M.L. is a thirty-four-year-old Bellport, New York, music teacher, married to a physical education instructor. Under his guidance, she has been working with weights specifically to build up her upper torso. She reported improved posture, increased muscular strength, and well-toned upper arms. "My increased strength has even improved my piano playing," she told Consumers Union. M.R., twenty-nine, of Chicago, wrote that she supplements "running by exercising with weights, which I have had at home for ten years. I can press sixty pounds easily, which is half my weight." She uses weights at least five days a week—"not long, just enough to increase my strength."

As these and many other women would attest, weight training does not lead to overmuscularization. The greater muscle mass in men is primarily the result of the male hormone testosterone. (This hormone is also present in women, but never at the level found in men.) Furthermore, the increase in strength that both men and women obtain from weight training is not entirely due to increased muscle size. To some extent it comes from an increase in the number of motor units (see page 84) activated during a muscle's contraction. If you use a weight training program to bring more muscles into play you can get a threefold increase in strength without getting a threefold increase in the size of your muscles. And once you develop your muscles to suit you, you can decrease the intensity of your workout (by decreasing the size of the weights, for example) to maintain rather than increase muscle size.

How does weight training affect body weight? Because weight training develops your muscles, it will increase the percentage of your body composition that is muscle.

Does this mean that somone interested in *reducing* body weight should avoid weight training? Not necessarily. To lose body fat—but not muscle—choose activities likely to burn plenty of calories if you sustain them over a long duration. If you jog, walk, swim, or bicycle, for example, you could count on losing weight over a period of time. If you supplement these activities with weight training, you will lose fat while gaining muscle.

If you want to *gain* weight, you should supplement your training program with a high-calorie diet. As your muscle size increases, your body weight will increase.

At what age can a youngster begin weight training? It's safe to begin weight training in early adolescence, as soon as a boy or girl shows interest in the activity. The idea that weight training can cause hernia, muscle-boundness, and heart damage has long been refuted. Quite the contrary. Controlled studies, including a study conducted by one of our senior authors with forty-six boys from twelve to seventeen years of age, have not shown any physical problems resulting from a program of weight training for young people.

Some youngsters may want to begin weight training when they see parents, older siblings, or friends enjoying benefits of muscle improvement— or just enjoying the activity of weight training itself. Others, like some of their elders, may be interested primarily in improving their musculature.

Many young people come to weight training to improve and maintain their strength and endurance in order to enhance their performance in competitive sports. Football players, gymnasts, runners, swimmers, and wrestlers often use weight training both in and out of season. An important advantage of weight training for younger as well as older athletes, in addition to improving sports performance, is the reduction of athletic injuries associated with improved muscular strength and endurance.

How old is too old for weight training? You're never too old for weight training. Healthy people in their fifties, sixties, seventies, or older can benefit from a sound weight training program, but it should be used to supplement a regimen emphasizing CRE activities such as walking, jogging, swimming, or bicycling.

Muscles often lose their strength with aging, but these losses can be minimized or reversed by regular weight training. The exercise, like any other, should be begun cautiously and increased slowly, especially by those who've been inactive. Beginning with light weights and few repetitions, older people can adjust gradually to the new activity. Weight training can be continued for as long as an older person is in reasonably good shape and has no cardiovascular problems.

Does exercise increase a woman's bust? Exercise cannot increase bust size, but it can strengthen the muscles supporting the breasts—and that can change appearance. To strengthen these muscles, a woman should select three or four exercises for the pectoral muscles, which are located on the front of the chest, and do the exercises for 8 to 15 repetitions every other day. (See chest exercises in the Glossary of Exercises.)

Calisthenics

Compared with weight training, calisthenics is less likely to help as much with muscular strength as with muscular endurance. But, push-ups, sit-ups, and other calisthenics can be used if weight training is not available or desirable.

If you can't do even a single push-up on the floor, begin a program in calisthenics by doing a push-up against the wall. (See the Glossary of Exercises.) Work up to 15 repetitions. Then work up to 15 repetitions using a table for support, and then switch to a chair. After that, you should be ready for the floor. At each stage you would use the three-set system—doing each set of repetitions three times every other day.

You can use an adjustable slant board as an aid in learning how to do sit-ups. Many nonathletes have mastered the sit-up by following this procedure. To begin, set the angle of elevation of the slant board fairly high. Position yourself on the slant board with your feet at the lower end. Try for a minimum of 6 repetitions and continue at that setting until you can do 15. Then lower the angle a bit and follow the same pattern of repetitions. Do this each time you lower the angle of the slant board until you can perform 15 sit-ups on a flat board. (Once again, use the three-set system for best results.)

Some cautions

Calisthenics, like weight training, is safe for those who qualify under our medical guidelines in Chapter 1. But, as we've said, people with coronary heart disease or coronary risk factors, circulatory problems, or hypertension should consult a physician before beginning such programs. The increase in blood pressure that occurs during the exercise program may be risky. And there are other cautions to observe as well.

Muscular training and orthopedic problems. Whether you rely on weight training or calisthenics to build up muscular strength and endurance, proceed cautiously if you have any orthopedic difficulties. Having orthopedic problems, however, does not mean that you must, as a matter of course, avoid exercise. If the problems are localized—and they usually are—an exercise program can be developed around them. If the difficulties involve specific groups of muscles, bones, or joints, it is usually possible to design a program that avoids using the affected part or parts while strengthening the rest of the body.

If, for example, you are recuperating from knee surgery, you can perform upper-body exercises while you sit or lie down. The other leg can also be exercised. Indeed, exercise programs are often designed specifically to rehabilitate orthopedic disabilities. Obviously, such a program must be designed with your individual problems in mind. Exercises that place too much strain on the lower back would simply aggravate a lower-back condition.

Consider J.L., a thirty-nine-year-old *Consumer Reports* reader from Mount Vernon, New York, who suffered month-long backaches on and off for several years. Finally his physician advised him to undertake weight training to strengthen his lower back. He went to a university gym for his specific therapeutic workout. While there, J.L. decided he might as well try a complete three-day-a-week program. He wrote that after three years, "I have progressed to a six-day-a-week split routine (three days on legs, chest, and back alternated with three days on arms, shoulders, and abdominals)." As for the original orthopedic difficulty, J.L. reported, "My back problems have gone away totally. . . . My original goal has been attained—no back pain."

No matter what your orthopedic condition, you should beware of lifting anything—whether a barbell or a suitcase—with your knees straight. Lifting from the floor should always be done with a straight back and bent knees, even by someone with no tendency to back weakness.

Exercises no one should do. Not all exercises are safe and sensible. Listed below are some to avoid no matter how much they may be touted as beneficial to you. Each of them may lead to injury.

■ The full squat, when performed repetitively, can injure knee ligaments. It includes among its variations repeated deep-knee bends, duck waddling, and the Russian bounce. These exercises have you squat low with the buttocks touching the back of the lower leg or the heels.

■ The straight leg sit-up, performed with legs extended and held straight, tends to pull the vertebrae forward. It increases the possibility of lordosis ("swayback"), a contributing factor to low-back problems. Be wary of this exercise, which is sometimes claimed to strengthen the abdominal muscles. The leg lift, also known as the leg raise, can cause some of the same problems as the straight leg sit-up.

Instead, do the bent knee sit-up, which places the workload more directly on the abdominal muscles. It is even more likely to do so if, when sitting up, you round your back until you reach the sit-up position.

■ In the straight-knee toe touch, you are supposed to bend over from a standing position, keeping your knees straight, and while bouncing try to touch the floor with your fingers. The back muscles would tend to be elongated, which would increase the possibility of "swayback" (see above).

■ The bent-over rowing motion falls into a different category. This exercise can be safe—and beneficial—if performed with the proper precautions. If done incorrectly, however, it can lead to injury. We recommend that you do the bent-over rowing motion (which you do while standing) only with your forehead resting on a table or some other support and your knees bent to ease the strain on the lower back.

"Negative" work and muscle soreness. Some exercise physiologists who have studied the "negative" phase of exercise—lowering yourself to the floor after pushing up, or lowering yourself after chinning up to a bar, or lowering to your chest a weight that you've lifted overhead—believe that it may contribute to muscle soreness. So-called negative work appears to be no less beneficial than the positive phase of exercise in contributing to training effects, although it is less fatiguing than positive exercise. But because of the possible association with muscle soreness, negative work should probably not be the primary focus of an exercise program.

A warning to weight lifters. One caution in particular should be observed by everyone who lifts weights. No matter how healthy you are, don't hold your breath during weight lifting. The rule is to inhale in preparation for the lift and exhale at the conclusion of the lift.

Even competitive weight lifters occasionally become light-headed from lifting an extremely heavy weight. The cause is a series of events, initiated during the lifting of weight, when a person tries to exhale with the epiglottis closed. (The epiglottis is a small flap of tissue deep in the throat; it prevents food or liquid from entering the windpipe.) The resulting increase in chest pressure activates the vagus nerve, which causes the heart to slow. That in turn may cause a drop in the blood flow to the brain to the point of light-headedness or even fainting.

Flexibility

The third musculoskeletal component of fitness is flexibility—the ability to flex and extend each joint through its normal range of motion. Flexibility in any joint depends on the condition of bones, tendons, ligaments, and muscles and on the interrelations of all these body parts.

Joints that are regularly moved through their full range of motion and muscles that regularly flex and extend fully will retain full normal mobility.

Flexibility is not a single characteristic uniformly present in all parts of the body. Some of your joints are probably a lot more flexible than others. Bursitis may limit the flexibility of your shoulder. Or bicycling may have improved the flexibility of your knees. To test your normal range of motion, you will need to move various joints in specified ways. The examples in Table 5-1 illustrate movements you can use to determine your flexibility for some of the important joints.

In the past it was believed that weight training could limit a person's flexibility and that strong people were likely to be muscle-bound. That myth has been laid to rest. Authorities now agree that flexibility is not impeded by weight training. In fact, champion weight lifters and body builders tend to be more flexible than average. It is true that activities that use only a limited range of motion in a particular muscle group may shorten the muscles involved. Jogging, for example, accentuates partial movements of muscle groups, and so encourages tightening of the hamstring muscles, the hip flexors (the muscles that bring the leg forward), and the quadriceps. But you can take steps to avoid the problem by supplementing your jogging with exercises designed to stretch those muscles. If you train with weights, you must be careful to keep your muscles flexible by performing each exercise correctly, moving through the full range of motion required. If you dance or do karate—exercises that promote flexibility—you probably already enjoy high levels of flexibility.

Regaining lost flexibility is a slow process, but well worth the time and effort. Persistence may pay off in marked improvement in flexibility. In working for flexibility, it's pointless to try to exceed the normal range of motion. In fact, extreme flexibility—loose-jointedness—is of no particular benefit and may even lead to stretched ligaments and weakness in some joints.

Anyone exercising to improve CRE or muscular fitness can benefit from flexibility training too. It is particularly well suited to the warm-up and cool-down periods. It can also help ease the pain and discomfort that may result from efforts to return to normal activity after an illness or a sedentary vacation. Flexibility training can also help overcome soreness after overdoing activities—overexertion on your first ski outing of the season, say. It can also help counter the ill-effects of sitting at a desk all day (shortening the hamstrings), wearing high-heeled shoes (shortening the Achilles tendon), or simply getting older.

A.D. from Bozeman, Montana, wrote that at age thirty-six, "I have to do regular stretching exercises to leave me flexible and decrease problems with tendinitis and lower-back aches and pains. After I learned about the need for flexibility exercise, I have performed it regularly (everyday) and

tried to do it right before handball, tennis, jogging, cycling, or skiing.
. . .The sessions only require about fifteen minutes or less."

The best way to develop flexibility is to use stretching exercises, and
the best way to stretch is slowly and gradually, using a technique called
static stretching. See stretching model program in Chapter 7.

Table 5–1

Normal Range of Joint Motion

This Table shows the normal range of motion for some of the major joints. By
comparing the motion of your joints with the illustrations below, you should be
able to determine whether you have normal range. The approximate degree of
movement is noted on each illustration. If any one of your joints has a limited
range, see stretching model program in Chapter 7. If you decide to try to increase
your range of motion, remember that for most people there is no need to achieve
flexibility beyond normal range.

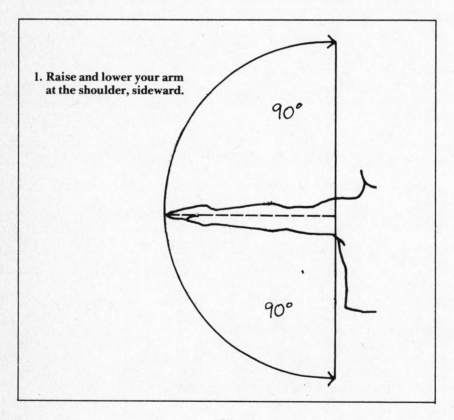

1. Raise and lower your arm
   at the shoulder, sideward.

90°

90°

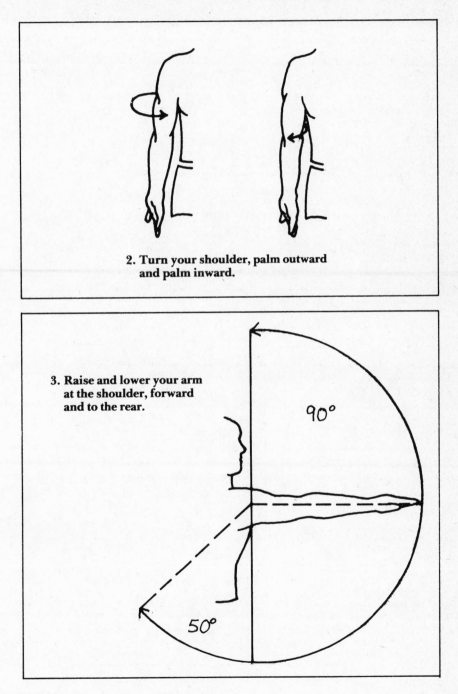

2. Turn your shoulder, palm outward and palm inward.

3. Raise and lower your arm at the shoulder, forward and to the rear.

90°

50°

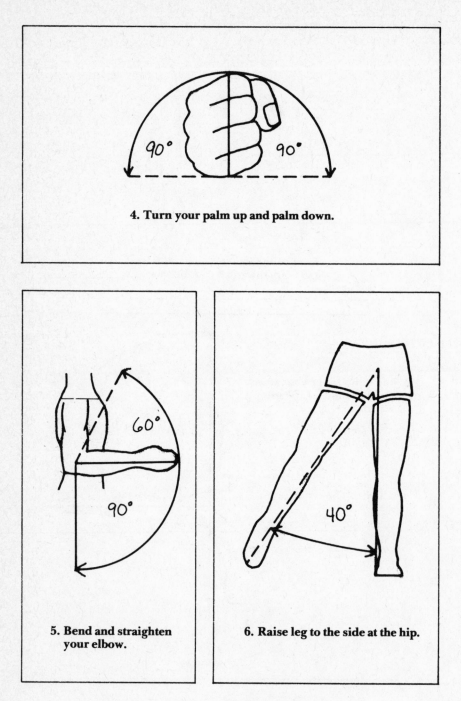

4. Turn your palm up and palm down.

5. Bend and straighten your elbow.

6. Raise leg to the side at the hip.

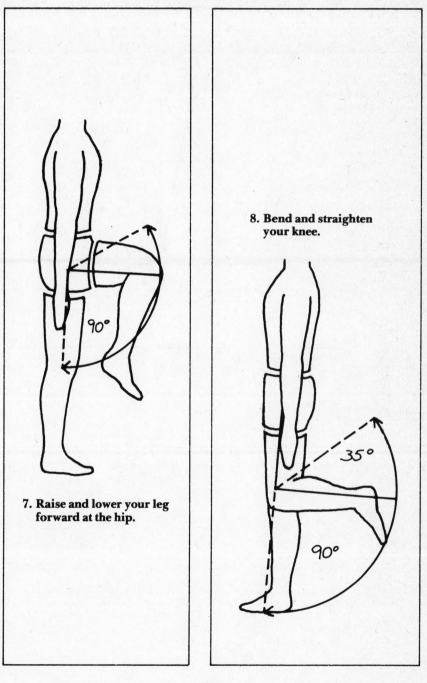

**8. Bend and straighten
your knee.**

90°

35°

90°

**7. Raise and lower your leg
forward at the hip.**

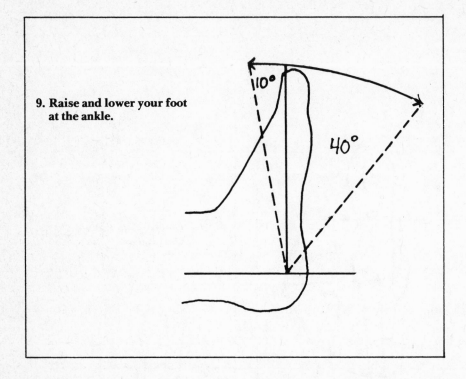

9. Raise and lower your foot at the ankle.

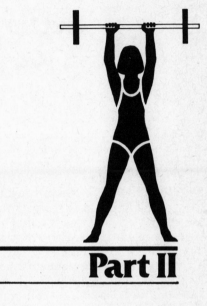

Part II

6

Getting Started
and Keeping Going

Even though you understand the theoretical basis of physical fitness, the importance of the five components, and the benefits you get from sports and other activities, you may still doubt your ability to stick with an exercise program. Perhaps you know from past experience or from your way of doing things that if you start an exercise program you may bog down, beg off, and finally quit. For those of you who are as apt to stop as you are to start, Chapter 6 offers suggestions to help you sustain your commitment to exercise.

This chapter presents five steps to help you get started on a fitness program—and to keep you going. Even if you think you're able to function well enough without a prescribed system, you may find all or some of these steps useful.

1. Setting goals

What do you hope to get out of your exercise program? To reduce your blood pressure? To "get some exercise" because your doctor told you to? To become stronger? To improve your looks? Or do you just think it will make you feel better? Knowing the goals you hope to accomplish by exercising can be an important first step in a successful program because it establishes the direction you want to go in. If you can resolve why you're starting to exercise, it can help you to keep going.

Table 1–18 on pages 43–44 lists a wide variety of potential goals. Studies have shown that many of these are indeed achievable by regular systematic exercise. Others are more general and the correlation between the benefits and exercise are often unproved. For example, a reduction in one's resting heart rate is easily and objectively measured and a predictable decrease can be a result of a cardiorespiratory endurance (CRE) program. Other goals, such as having more energy at the end of the day, are more subjective and cannot be as readily measured. Even though some exercisers may not achieve all their goals, they will still get benefits.

In Chapter 1 you were asked to assess your current fitness level and determine which fitness components need improvement. You were then asked to identify the goals that you wish to achieve through exercise. If you have not yet set your goals, do so now before you decide on a specific exercise program.

2. Selecting a sport or activity

The success of your exercise program could depend on the activity you select. A fitness program requires a commitment. And you're more likely to stick to it if you choose an interesting and pleasurable program. The right program will increase your incentive to continue. The wrong program becomes drudgery—a chore that you will eventually hate to do.

Chapter 7 offers a variety of model programs that can get you started. Chapter 8 describes sports and activities, providing information about them. Try to select a number of sports or activities. Variety can help avoid boredom as well as let you put together a year-round program. For example, you may enjoy winter sports, but if your exercise is then limited to just a few months, your fitness level will also be limited unless you supplement your program with other activities. If your favotite activities are all for the outdoors, it may be wise to select some indoor alternatives for bad-weather days. Whatever you do, don't decide impulsively on any exercise program. Take into consideration the points discussed below.

Your fitness needs

As you know from Chapter 2, one of the basic principles of sound fitness training is specificity—matching your activities to your goals. If you want, say, to improve your circulation, you need to select activities with high CRE benefits, such as aerobic dance, bicycling, jogging, rope skipping, swimming, or walking. To eliminate or reduce low-back pain, you need such activities as weight training and calisthenics to develop muscular strength, muscular endurance, and flexibility. If you're interested in overall improvement, then you should select activities in which you can develop all five fitness components.

Don't commit yourself to an activity just because it seems to meet your fitness needs. Check it out first. Is the activity enjoyable? Not an easy question to answer. In selecting activities, limit yourself to those that at least seem to be fun and that interest you. Don't select an activity just because it's the "in" thing. Chances are if you stick to what appeals to you, you're going to honor your commitment.

Health, skill, and fitness

Some people have health problems that either direct them toward a specific sport or activity because it is beneficial, or direct them away because it is contraindicated. (A number of health problems are discussed in Chapter 11.)

Some sports and activities require such a high level of skill that they are not a practical choice for beginners starting a fitness program. You may not have the ability, time, or interest to become proficient enough in a particular sport or activity to use it as a vehicle for fitness.

Your current fitness level sets limits of its own. For example, if you have low CRE, it would be unwise to start a jogging program: A walking program would be a more appropriate way to begin exercising. Unless you are very fit, select activities that are self-paced at first so that you can control the intensity and the duration. Competitive sports, for instance, could overtax many sedentary people.

Age

Older exercisers can participate in many activities but should think twice about activities that require high levels of speed, movement, reaction time, and other qualities of motor ability. Unless these skills have been maintained over the years, such activities are not recommended. (The question of sports and older people is discussed in Chapter 10.)

Convenience

Convenience covers a multitude of things to consider: availability of special facilities, location of the exercise site, time needed to get there, dependence on weather conditions, the need for other participants, and seasonal nature of the activity. You also need to consider carefully how you will find time to exercise. Unless exercise fits easily into your daily schedule, it's unlikely that you will continue your program.

Cost

Some sports and activities require equipment, fees, or membership investments that may strain the budget. Yet, there is no relationship between the fitness benefits of an activity and what it may cost. If money is an important consideration, limit your choice to activities that are inexpensive or even free. Remember that your selection may be temporary, so avoid a large financial investment until you're sure it's going to work out well.

Social aspects

The social potential of a sport or an activity can be a double-edged sword. On the one hand, if other people are needed, you may have a problem whenever they are not available. On the other hand, having others available can be a powerful incentive to get started and keep going.

When you consider all these criteria and narrow your choices, you will find yourself establishing priorities and juggling the variables. You may end up selecting an activity because it's convenient and does what you want it to do within the time you have available, rather than because it's fun or interesting. Remember that selections are temporary and can be changed. So once again, try to avoid any large outlay of money until you are sure of your choices.

3. Making a commitment

To change your exercise behavior, you have to make a deal with yourself—not just count on good intentions. This time make a deal in the form of a written contract. The contract should clearly state what you are going to do, why you want to do it, when you're going to start, the specific goals you expect to achieve, and the specific time you set for meeting the goals. A carefully designed contract can help to convert your good intentions—and vague aspirations that encourage excuses and delays—to clear, detailed procedures that promote action. By putting it in writing, you make a firm commitment—and you may be more likely to carry through to your goal.

Table 6–1 is a sample contract to use as a guide. (Before you fill out a contract, you may need to look through Chapters 7 and 8 to decide which programs or activities are for you.) After identifying the fitness goals you wish to achieve and listing them at the top of the contract, you are ready to apply the training principles of progressive overload and specificity. (Specificity means you select the activity specific to the goals; progressive overload is determined by intensity, duration, and frequency.)

It is likely that you can achieve your goals only after you stick to your exercise program for a long time. Because that's the case, it's usually helpful to state short-range goals. As they are accomplished, you can declare new short-range goals. Continue the process until you reach your long-range goals and have achieved the fitness benefits you are seeking.

4. Beginning and maintaining your program

Always start out doing less than you think you can, and progress slowly until you meet your goals. Give your body time to accept the change—something particularly important for sports and activities that require muscular adjustments. Don't let your initial enthusiasm trick you into exceeding your capacity. Be realistic, be patient—results take time.

The following guidelines may help you to get started and keep going.

■ Make your activity an unconditional part of your daily or weekly schedule. Set aside a regular time for exercise, and resist all efforts and temptations to deter you. Choose the time that fits your schedule, even though you may not always be at your best at that hour. Set aside *adequate* time: Allow for a proper ten-minute warm-up, a cool-down, and a shower (see stretching model program in Chapter 7).

■ Take advantage of whatever exercise opportunities present themselves: Walk to work, to the station or bus stop, up and down stairs—every chance you get.

■ Do what you can to avoid boredom. When you use a stationary bicycle or rowing machine at home, you might watch TV, listen to music,

---

Table 6–1

Sample Contract

I _____ am contracting with myself to follow an exercise program to achieve the following fitness goals.

    1. Increase resistance to fatigue

    2. Improve fit of clothes

    3. Lower the resting heart rate

    4. Become more muscular

    5. _____.

I will begin my program on _____. It will consist of the following:

Fitness components	Short-range goals	Exercise commitments
CRE Jogging/running (See model program in Chapter 7)	Jog 30 minutes within EBZ in one month	Work out every other day
Body composition Walking (See model program in Chapter 7)	Lose 8 pounds in 8 weeks	Walk briskly on nonjogging days for a minimum of 30 minutes
Muscular strength and endurance Weight training (See model program in Chapter 7)	Increase 30 percent in both muscular strength and endurance in 6 weeks	Do 3 sets of 8 to 15 repetitions every other day

I agree to maintain a record of my activity, assess my progress periodically, and, if necessary, revise my goals.

Signed _____   Date _____

or read (with the help of a music stand). Some joggers use headphones to listen to music (but don't do it near automobile traffic—that could be dangerous). And calisthenics at home can be done to music.

■ Exercising with others can be useful. But try to keep the group to no more than three or four. And try also to form a group that shares your goals and is at your level of competence.

■ Vary the program. Change the activity periodically—alone or with a group. If walking, jogging, or bicycling, change the route or the distance every now and then. Racquet sport enthusiasts might find it adds interest to change partners after a while or to try a new location.

5. Recording and assessing progress

Recording and assessing your progress after each exercise session— whether you make progress or not—can help you keep track of how you're doing. A record that notes the daily results of your program will give you a sense of accomplishment and remind you of your commitment.

Take a look at the sample progress chart (see Table 6–2) to get some ideas about how you might set up your own weekly record system. For a sample of a daily record system, see Table 7–10 on page 129. No matter what form your record takes, keep it handy and post the results immediately after each exercise session.

If this strikes you as rigid, you're right. But remember that the main reason you're doing it is to help you get started and keep going. Stay with the record-keeping and give yourself enough time to begin to experience rewards. Once you've achieved your short-range goals, you'll discover less resistance to exercising—and a more favorable attitude toward the commitment to exercise.

There are no hard and fast rules to tell you how quickly you should progress. If you're doing a CRE activity, however, your heart rate can serve as your guide (see page 62).

In the first few weeks, you may find that the goals you have set are unrealistic. If so, upgrade or downgrade the goals in your contract. If you find that your selection of activities has not been successful, switch to some other form of exercise. Expect this initial experience to be experimental, with many adjustments and changes.

Don't expect progress to be even and regular. On some days you'll feel good and your progress will be outstanding. But on other days, you'll barely be able to perform. These fluctuations are quite common—don't be concerned.

Don't rush yourself. Proceed slowly and increase your work load gradually. Your program is not for a week or a month, but for a lifetime. With a long way to go, there's no need for overzealousness, which can result in injury or enough discomfort to discourage your continued participation.

Table 6–2

Weekly Log for CRE Program

This is a sample progress chart on which you can record the distance covered or the time spent for each day of the week on a CRE activity. (Calories are taken from Table 7–4.) You can adapt this log to use for more than one activity.

Week	Activities	Daily distance or time							Weekly distance or time	Weekly calorie cost
		Mon.	Tues.	Wed.	Thur.	Fri.	Sat.	Sun.		
1	Walking	30 min.		30 min.		30 min.		30 min.	2 hrs.	468
2	Walking		30 min.	30 min.	30 min.		30 min.	30 min.	2 hrs. 30 min.	585
3	Walk/jog		35 min.	35 min.		35 min.		35 min.	2 hrs. 20 min.	882
4										
5										
6										
7										
8										
9										
10										
11										

7

Model Programs

By showing you how to get started and by setting reasonable standards for performance, a model program can launch you effectively into exercise and keep you going. It gives you a structured way to apply progressive overload and specificity—the two key training principles. If you stick with a model program, your fitness is bound to improve.

If you're fit enough to exercise, you're qualified to start a model program. None of them requires more than entry-level skills. You would not need any special sports ability or experience to begin a model program. Chances are you can find one in this chapter that demands little more in the way of athletic skills than those you have already.

Choosing a model program

Your task now is to select the appropriate program from among the eight basic models presented in this chapter. Our senior authors have developed these models based on their experience designing regimens to meet almost every kind of fitness goal and to strengthen all of the fitness components. The eight prototypes presented here have been fully tested and have been shown to give realistic results.

Thus your problem is not deciding whether a particular model program is likely to be effective, but rather which one is going to be right for you. To choose a model program, begin by reviewing your specific fitness goals (see Table 1–18, pages 43–44). That should be your starting point. Using Table 1–18, you can tie in your fitness goals to the fitness components involved in achieving them. Then turn to Table 7–1 to find out which model programs are likely to benefit the particular components on which you have to concentrate to attain your fitness goals.

Next, narrow your choice. Read through the descriptions of the programs you're considering and decide which model will work best for you. Your final selection should be a program that adapts well to your present routine, seems enjoyable, and sounds like something you can start without major changes in your life-style. Avoid a time-consuming regimen if you're already overscheduled. Or if the early morning will be your time to exercise and you tend to wake up cranky and untalkative, stick to a simple program that can be followed in splendid isolation.

Agreed, no model program is likely to change you very much during the first few weeks of exercise. But what if the exercise program you chose

---

Table 7–1

Relating Model Programs to Fitness Components

For each model program listed below, a rating of high (H), moderate (M), or low (L) indicates the extent to which the program benefits each of the five components of physical fitness.

Model program	Components of Physical Fitness				
	Cardio-respiratory endurance	Body composition	Muscular strength*	Muscular endurance*	Flexibility*
Walking/jogging/running	H	H	M	H	L
Interval circuit training	H	H	H	H	M
Calisthenic circuit training	H	H	M	H	M
Stretching (warm-up/cool-down)	L	L	L	L	H
Bicycling	H	H	M	H	M
Rope skipping	H	H	M	H	L
Swimming	H	H	M	H	M
Weight training	L	M	H	H	H

---

*Ratings for these components are based on benefits for the specific muscle groups used during the activity in question. (See description of exercises for these model programs in this chapter to identify the muscle groups benefited.) For all other muscle groups, the rating would be low (L).

does not seem suitable after you try it for a reasonable time. All may not be lost. It's possible that you can make adjustments in a model program to adapt it to your particular needs. But give the program a chance: Don't be too hasty about making changes. For three to four weeks, follow faithfully the specifics of the model program you chose. Then if you do decide to adapt the regimen so it becomes more suited to your likes and dislikes, be sure you retain the basic elements of the program. For example, you may decide to change the specific exercises in the interval circuit training model program, but keep the system intact. Don't change the amount of time specified for exercise or rest.

Walking/jogging/running

Walking, jogging, and running are the most popular options for those who want to improve cardiorespiratory endurance (CRE) and body composition. Exercise on foot is by far the most common form of CRE training in the United States. These days there may be as many as 17 million people who jog regularly. And millions more, particularly those over sixty, walk as their favorite form of exercise. Walking, jogging, and running require no special skills, expensive equipment, or unusual facilities. Comfortable clothing, well-fitted walking or running shoes, and a stopwatch or ordinary watch with a second hand are all you need. What's more, like most CRE activities, they are effective techniques for weight control and changing body composition. They will also improve muscular endurance of the legs.

It's not always easy to distinguish among these three forms of CRE activities. Walking may vary from a 2-mile-per-hour pace that is leisurely for most people but may be taxing for others to a 9-mile-per-hour competitive pace that is faster than some can jog or run. When the pace is between 7 and 8 miles per hour, it's just as hard to tell where jogging ends and running begins. For clarity and consistency, we will consider *walking* any on-foot exercise of less than 5 miles per hour, *jogging* any pace between 5 and 7.5 miles per hour, and *running* any pace faster than that.

Table 7–2 divides walking, jogging, and running into nine categories with rates of speed and calorie costs for each. As you see, these activities can use a relatively large number of calories per minute. The faster your pace or the longer you exercise, the more calories you burn. The greater the amount of calories burned, the higher the potential effectiveness of these activities for developing and maintaining CRE, improving body composition, and losing weight. Singly or in any combination, walking, jogging, or running can be done briskly enough to keep your heart rate within the exercise benefit zone (EBZ) long enough to burn a large number of calories each session. (See pages 62–66 for a discussion of EBZ.) By gradually increasing the total number of calories used, you can progress to a level of fitness required for you to achieve your goals. Once

Table 7–2

Walking/Jogging/Running

This Table gives the calorie costs of walking, jogging, and running for a slow, moderate, and fast pace. Calculations for calorie costs are based on calories per minute per pound. They are approximate and assume a level terrain. A hilly terrain would result in higher calorie cost. Use this method to get an estimate of the number of calories you burn: Multiply your weight by the calories per minute per pound (listed in the right-hand column) for the speed at which you're doing the activity.

Activity	Speed		Calories per minute per pound
	Miles per hour	Minutes:seconds per mile	
Walking			
Slow	2.0	30:00	.020
	2.5	24:00	.023
Moderate	3.0	20:00	.026
	3.5	17:08	.029
Fast	4.0	15:00	.037
	4.5	13:20	.048
Jogging			
Slow	5.0	12:00	.060
	5.5	11:00	.074
Moderate	6.0	10:00	.081
	6.7	9:00	.088
Fast	7.0	8:35	.092
	7.5	8:00	.099
Running			
Slow	8.5	7:00	.111
Moderate	9.0	6:40	.116
Fast	10.0	6:00	.129
	11.0	5:30	.141

you achieve the fitness level you set as your goal, you can occasionally ease up a bit on intensity and duration, and reduce frequency.

The five variations of the basic walking/jogging/running model program that follow are designed to help you regulate the intensity, duration, and frequency of your program. To select the particular model that's best for you at your current CRE level, consult Table 7–3.

General guidelines for a walking/jogging/running program

Here are some guidelines to help you make whichever one of the five model programs you select an effective training regimen. (Also see Chapter 12 for information on related matters, including shoes and clothing.)

EBZ and heart rate. To measure progress with any of these model programs, you will need to know how to take your pulse (see page 64) and how to determine your EBZ. All five walking/jogging/running model programs are based on raising heart rate into the EBZ. To work effectively for CRE training or to improve body composition, you may need to adjust your pace as you increase in fitness. Monitor your pulse to find out if your heart rate is in your EBZ.

Intensity. Begin *very* slowly if you're a novice at exercise or used to a sedentary life-style. Give your muscles a chance to adjust to the increased work load. At the outset, it may be wise to keep your heart rate below the EBZ until your body has had time to adapt to new demands.

Even if you're not a beginner, you may find you're going at a slow pace because at first you may not need to walk or jog very fast to keep your heart rate in the EBZ. As your CRE improves, however, you will probably need to increase intensity. As you progress in CRE, chances are that you not only will pick up the pace automatically, but you may discover you don't even need to take your pulse to find out if your heart rate is in your EBZ. For one thing, if you exercise with a friend, you can rely on the "talk test"—the ability to keep up a conversation comfortably during exercise.

Duration and frequency. To experience training effects, we recommend a minimum of fifteen minutes of exercise within the EBZ each session for model programs 2 through 5. Frequency of exercise should be three times a week—more often if your goal includes changing body composition or losing weight.

Interval training. Some of the model programs involve continuous activity; others rely on interval training, which calls for alternating a relief interval with exercise (walking after you jog, say). Interval training can prolong the total time you spend in exercise and delay the onset of fatigue. A *set* is a combination of an exercise interval and a relief (or rest) interval.

111

Table 7–3

Selecting a Walking/Jogging/Running Model Program

Model program 1: walking (starting)

Choose this program if *any* of the following apply:
- You have medical restrictions.
- You are recovering from illness or surgery.
- You tire easily after short walks.
- You are 50 pound or more overweight.
- You have a sedentary life-style.

And if you want to prepare for the advanced walking program (see below) to improve CRE, body composition, and muscular endurance.

Model program 2: walking (advanced)

Choose this program if:
- You already can walk comfortably for 30 minutes.

And if you want to develop and maintain cardiorespiratory fitness, a lean body, and muscular endurance.

Model program 3: walking/jogging (starting)

Choose this program if:
- You already can walk comfortably for 30 minutes.

And if you want to prepare for the jogging/running program (see below) to improve CRE, body composition, and muscular endurance.

Model program 4: jogging/running

Choose this program if both of the following apply:
- You already can jog comfortably without muscular discomfort.
- You already can jog for 15 minutes within your EBZ without stopping or for 30 minutes with brief walking intervals.

And if you want to develop and maintain a high level of cardiorespiratory fitness, a lean body, and muscular endurance.

Model program 5: running (racing)

Choose this program if *all* of the following apply:
- You already can jog/run comfortably within your EBZ for 30 to 60 minutes.
- You have been jogging/running regularly for at least 3 months.
- You have had a stress test (if you are among those for whom one is recommended—see page 59).

And if you want to train for road races as a way of maintaining a high level of cardiorespiratory fitness, a lean body, and muscular endurance.

Warm-up and cool-down. No matter which one of the walking/jogging/running model programs you select, always begin each exercise session with a ten-minute warm-up. (See warm-up/cool-down in stretching model program.) This will help prevent loss of flexibility, which could be caused by the limited range of motion in walking/jogging/running. Avoid an abrupt transition from the warm-up phase to the active portion of your workout. To extend the warm-up period, begin your walk, jog, or run at a slower than usual pace to the point where you can maintain your workout within the EBZ. As you're ending your exercise session, always slow down gradually to bring your system back to its normal state. In addition to cooling down, it's a good idea to repeat the stretching exercises that were part of your warm-up.

Record-keeping. It's important to keep track of how you do on a walk/jog/run program. After each exercise session, record your daily distance (or time) on a progress chart, set up to show your weekly totals (see Table 6–2, page 106). At the end of each week, enter the total distance (or time) for the week and the total amount of calories expended in your exercise sessions.

Model program 1: walking (starting)

Purpose: To prepare for the advanced walking program to improve CRE, body composition, and muscular endurance.

Intensity. Start at 50 to 60 percent of estimated maximum heart rate (MHR), which is below your EBZ. (See page 62 for a discussion of how to calculate MHR and EBZ.) Gradually increase your pace, still keeping below your EBZ.

Duration. Walk at first for fifteen minutes at a comfortable pace. Gradually increase to thirty-minute sessions. Distance will vary from one to two miles.

Frequency. At the beginning, walk every other day. Gradually increase to daily walking if your purpose includes achieving a lean body.

Calorie cost. Work up to using about 90 to 135 calories in each session. (See Table 7–4.)

Progression. Once your muscles have become adjusted to the exercise program, increase the duration of your sessions—but no more than 10 percent a week. Increase your intensity only enough to keep your heart rate just below your EBZ When you're able to walk one and a half miles in thirty minutes, using from 90 to 135 calories per session, you should consider moving on to conditioning yourself to a maintenance walking program—model program 2: walking (advanced)—or to model program 3: walking/jogging (starting).

At the beginning

Start the walking model program at whatever level you feel comfortable. Maintain a normal easy pace and stop to rest as often as you need to.

113

Table 7–4

Determining Calorie Cost Using Model Programs 1, 2, and 3

This Table gives the approximate calorie costs per pound of body weight of walking or walking/jogging from 15 minutes to 60 minutes for distances of .50 mile up to 5.25 miles at varying rates of speed. These calorie costs are based on walking or jogging on a level terrain. To use the Table, find on the horizontal line the approximate length of time you walk or jog. Then locate on the vertical column the approximate distance you cover. The figure at the intersection represents an estimate of the calories used per pound of body weight.* Multiply this figure by your own body weight to get the total number of calories used. For example, assuming you weigh 135 pounds and walk 3.50 miles in 60 minutes, you would burn 235 calories: 1.74 (calories per pound, from Table) × 135 (weight) = 235 calories.

Distance (in miles)	Time (in minutes)									
	15	20	25	30	35	40	45	50	55	60
.50	.30									
.75	.39	.43	.47							
1.00	.56	.52	.56	.60						
1.25	.90	.63	.65	.69						
1.50	1.20	.96	.74	.78	.82					
1.75	1.39	1.32	1.03	.87	.91	.95	.99			
2.00		1.61	1.38	1.11	1.00	1.04	1.08	1.12		
2.25		1.79	1.78	1.44	1.18	1.13	1.17	1.21	1.25	1.29
2.50			2.01	1.81	1.47	1.27	1.26	1.30	1.34	1.38
2.75			2.19	2.23	1.85	1.57	1.35	1.39	1.43	1.47
3.00			2.37	2.41	2.22	1.92	1.67	1.48	1.52	1.56
3.25				2.59	2.63	2.23	1.96	1.76	1.61	1.65
3.50					2.81	2.65	2.29	2.06	1.83	1.74
3.75						3.03	2.71	2.39	2.08	1.90
4.00						3.21	3.10	2.76	2.41	2.23
4.25							3.43	3.15	2.78	2.50
4.50							3.61	3.57	3.18	2.87
4.75								3.83	3.51	3.19
5.00								4.01	3.96	3.62
5.25									4.23	3.97

*Because rapid walking and jogging are less efficient than slow and moderate walking, you burn more calories at a shorter duration than you burn over a longer period even though the distance covered is the same.

114

Walk the routes you enjoy—and be on the lookout for pleasant new routes for walks.

From the beginning, try to walk every other day, even if the walk lasts only a few minutes. Never prolong a walk past the point of comfort. If you overdo, you're likely to end up with sore muscles and maybe even injuries —the path to becoming an "exercise drop-out."

Walking with a friend may help to keep you going, so try to persuade one to join you. When walking with a friend, let a comfortable conversation be your guide to pace.

One *Consumer Reports* reader, H.G., age sixty-eight, of Merrillville, Indiana, wrote he had begun his walking program ten years earlier, after a heart attack put him in the hospital. Four weeks after the heart attack, H.G. began walking a few minutes each day. Gradually, he extended his walking and in time was up to two miles a day. He now walks "at a good clip," covering two miles in thirty minutes. Bad weather doesn't stop him: He walks in his large basement. His walking program is "all in all a tremendous benefit," brightening his outlook, increasing energy for work around the house, and leading to new friends.

As you progress

Don't be discouraged by lack of immediate progress. And don't try to speed things up by overdoing, especially if your life has been sedentary. The change to a schedule of regular slow-paced walking will be sufficient to improve your CRE.

Soon you may be walking for a longer time than usual and taking fewer and shorter rest stops. You may feel instinctively when it would be comfortable to pick up the pace. As you approach your target of a comfortable thirty-minute walk, you may be able to increase your rate of speed enough so that you approach the lower level of your EBZ (70 percent of your MHR). The pace at which different people walk in order to reach 70 percent of estimated MHR can vary considerably. For some, it will be a slow 2 miles per hour. For others, it will be a moderate 3.5 miles per hour. Of course, pace and heart rate can vary with the terrain, the weather, and other factors.

Measuring calories

Suppose you begin this model program with a fifteen-minute walk for one-half mile. A look at Table 7–4 will show that if you weigh 154 pounds you would have burned 46 calories. If you walk double the distance in just a few more minutes, you will almost double the number of calories used. But the rate of speed would also have to double and that pace may be too taxing for anyone whose beginning CRE dictated selection of this model program. Instead, you should aim to increase calorie costs by walking for a longer time or for a longer distance rather than by increasing your rate of speed.

Model program 2: walking (advanced)

Purpose: To develop and maintain cardiorespiratory fitness, a lean body, and muscular endurance.

Intensity. Start at a pace within your EBZ but soon begin to walk at a little faster pace. This might boost your heart rate into the upper levels of your EBZ, which is fine for brief periods. But don't overdo the intervals of fast walking. Slow down after a short time to drop your pulse rate. Gradually, you can lengthen the periods of fast walking and shorten the relief intervals of slow walking. Vary your regimen to allow for intervals of slow, medium, and fast walking.

Duration. Walk at first for thirty minutes. Gradually increase your walking time until eventually you reach sixty minutes, all the while keeping within your EBZ. Distance will vary from two to four miles.

Frequency. Walk every other day. Exercise more frequently if your purpose includes changing body composition.

Calorie cost. Work up to using about 200 to 350 calories in each session. (See Table 7–4.)

Progression. As your heart rate adjusts to the increased work load, gradually increase your pace and your total walking time. Interval training (see page 126) is an effective way to achieve progressive overload: When your heart rate gets too high, slow down to lower your pulse rate until you're at the low end of your EBZ. Eventually, you will reach the fitness level you would like to maintain. For some, it may be the ability to walk at a rapid 4 miles per hour for thirty minutes; for others, it may be a more leisurely walk extending over sixty minutes or longer. To maintain the level of fitness you choose for yourself, continue to burn the same amount of calories as you did to reach that fitness level.

At the beginning

Begin the advanced walking program by keeping within your familiar thirty-minute walking time but walk somewhat faster. Check your pulse to make sure you keep your heart rate within your EBZ. Slow down when necessary to lower your heart rate when going up hills or when extending the duration of your walks. Using this form of interval training, gradually you will be able to extend the periods of faster walking and decrease the number and length of the relief intervals of slow walking. In time, you will be able to walk for longer than thirty minutes and at a faster pace as your CRE level improves, with your heart rate remaining comfortably within your EBZ.

J.E., a thirty-eight-year-old woman from Asheville, North Carolina, decided that for her busy schedule of teaching and household responsibilities, brisk walking would be the way to get in shape and stay in shape. She told Consumers Union that she started with a daily mile and gradually worked up to four miles. Once she reached 4 miles per hour at a moderate-to-fast pace she was able to maintain her fitness level even though she skips a day or two or cuts back from a walk of four miles to three.

At her low weight of 98 pounds, J.E. uses about 219 calories during each sixty-minute session. In a typical week of daily walking, she does more than 1,500 calories worth of exercise, a total that apparently played a part in altering her body composition. J.E. reported that she has lost one to two inches each from her waist, hips, and thighs and was maintaining her 5-foot frame in this condition. J.E. credits her regular walking program with helping her eliminate midafternoon fatigue, sleep well at night, and feel comfortable enough to stop taking four tranquilizers a day—a habit of sixteen years. What's more, J.E. wrote, "My walk is my thinking/problem-solving time."

As you progress

Vary your regimen by changing the pace and distance walked or by walking routes with different terrains and views. Some days, too, you may have only limited time for exercise. If your usual workout consists of a leisurely 3-mile-per-hour walk that takes sixty minutes, try the following variations if you need to save time and still keep your exercise schedule: Increase your intensity to as much as 4.5 miles per hour and decrease your duration and distance by walking two and a quarter miles in thirty minutes. Don't use this option, however, if by speeding up your pace you move your heart rate beyond your EBZ for longer than brief periods.

As you progress, maintain your heart rate within your EBZ. Do not, as a regular practice, keep your pulse high for more than brief periods. Although picking up the pace can burn more calories per minute, it also promotes fatigue—thus tending to limit the duration of the session. In the end, you could be burning fewer calories. Make use of interval training with its regulated control of pace to maintain your heart rate at a desired level. It also introduces variety into a continuous walking program done at the same pace—a monotonous prospect for some.

Measuring calories

Table 7–4 will help you assess the calorie benefits of time spent doing model program 2. Use the table to give direction to your sessions and to gauge progress toward whatever calorie goal you've set.

Model program 3: walking/jogging (starting)

Purpose: To prepare for the jogging/running program to improve CRE, body composition, and muscular endurance.

Intensity. Start by walking at a moderate pace (3 to 4 miles per hour). Staying within your EBZ, begin to add brief intervals of slow jogging (5 to 6 miles per hour). Keep the walking intervals constant at sixty seconds or at 110 yards. Gradually increase the jogging intervals.

Duration. Each exercise session should last fifteen to thirty minutes, alternating walking with jogging. Eventually, your time spent jogging will be at least four times as long as for walking. Distances will vary from one and a half to two and a half miles.

Frequency. Exercise every other day. Exercise more frequently by walking only, on days you're not walking/jogging, if your purpose includes changing body composition.

Calorie cost. Work up to using about 200 to 350 calories in each session. (See Table 7–4.)

Progression. Choose the walking/jogging progression that suits you best—either one based on time (see Table 7–5) or distance (see Table 7–6). Adjust your ratio of walking to jogging as you increase your jogging to keep within your EBZ as much as possible. When you have progressed to the point where most of your thirty-minute session is spent jogging, you should consider moving on to model program 4: jogging/running.

Even after you move on to model program 4, you will find it useful to go back to walking/jogging, perhaps combined with features of the jogging/running program, as an effective way to maintain high levels of fitness.

At the beginning

Start the walking/jogging program slowly. Until your muscles adjust to jogging, you may need to exercise at less than your EBZ. At the outset,

---

Table 7–5

Sample Walking/Jogging Progression by Time

This Table is based on a walking interval of 3.75 miles per hour, measured in seconds, and a jogging interval of 5.5 miles per hour, measured in minutes: seconds. The combination of the two intervals equals a single set. Under the heading "Number of sets," the higher figure represents the maximum number of sets to be completed.

Walk interval (seconds)	Jog interval (minutes:seconds)	Number of sets	Total distance (miles)	Total time (minutes: seconds)
:60	:30	10–15	1.0–1.7	15:00–22:30
:60	:60	8–13	1.2–2.0	16:00–26:00
:60	2:00	5–19	1.3–2.3	15:00–27:00
:60	3:00	5–7	1.6–2.4	16:00–28:00
:60	4:00	3–6	1.5–2.7	15:00–30:00

expect to do two to four times as much walking as jogging. If you're relatively inexperienced at jogging and find your heart rate is consistently at the top of your EBZ or above it, you may need to do even more walking than that. Be guided by how comfortable you feel—and by your heart rate—in setting the pace for your progress. At first, check your heart rate often. In time you should develop a sense of when you're in your EBZ. But don't overdo: Limit your progress to weekly increments of not more than 10 percent in intensity or duration.

A.K.J., a mid-Manhattan dweller in her fifties, began a walk/jog program at her physician's suggestion. She described herself to Consumers Union as having become "rather flabby and generally out of shape" with various medical problems. Already accustomed to walking extensively, A.K.J. took a stress test before beginning a jogging program "to be on the safe side." Her program consisted of eight weeks of brisk walking for at least thirty minutes (or one and a half or two miles) three to four times a week. In the second eight weeks, A.K.J. began jogging on a two-to-one ratio (two parts walk to one part jog). She confesses to having been "a total flop" at taking her pulse as she increased the level of exercise because she never learned to "distinguish between the beat of my pulse and the noises around me."

A.K.J.'s exercise regimen and a careful diet combined to do away with "most of the flab (17 pounds worth)." Running on city sidewalks, however, contributed to "painful knee problems" as did, perhaps, a

---

Table 7–6

Sample Walking/Jogging Progression by Distance

This Table is based on a walking interval of 3.75 miles per hour, measured in yards, and a jogging interval of 5.5 miles per hour, also measured in yards. The combination of the two intervals equals a single set.

Walk interval (yards)	Jog interval (yards)	Number of sets	Total distance (miles)	Total time (minutes: seconds)
110	55	11–21	1.0–2.0	15:00–28:12
110	110	16	2.0	26:56
110	220	11	2.0	26:02
110	330	8	2.0	24:24
110	440	7	2.2	26:05
110	440	8	2.5	29:49

tendency on A.K.J.'s part to give short shrift to her warm-up exercises.

As you progress

Like A.K.J. once she phased into jogging, you may have started on a two-to-one ratio. Assume your plan is to progress to a one-to-four ratio —one part walk to four parts jog. (The number of sets—the combinations of exercise and relief intervals—that you do in an exercise session may range from three to twenty-one.) To make it easier to organize your workouts and to measure progress, keep the walking interval constant at sixty seconds or 110 yards as you gradually increase the jogging interval. You may complete anywhere from one mile to more than two and a half miles within fifteen to thirty minutes.

To find a walking/jogging progression that suits you, refer to Tables 7–5 and 7–6. (One uses time, the other distance.) Which one you choose will depend, to some extent, on where you work out. If you have access to a track or can use a measured distance with easily visible landmarks to indicate yardage covered, you may find it convenient to use distance as your organizing principle. If you'll be using parks, streets, or woods, time intervals (measured with a watch) would probably work better.

The suggested progressions in Tables 7–5 and 7–6—by time or distance—are not meant to be rigid mandates. Rather, they embody guidelines to help you develop your own rate of progress. The Tables are based on a pace of 3.75 miles per hour for walking and of 5.5 miles per hour for jogging, but don't be bound by that: Adjust your tempo to what suits you best. For some people, the recommended beginning two-to-one ratio or the suggested rate of speed may be too low or too high. No matter which method you follow, let your progress be guided by your heart rate. Increase intensity and duration only to get your heart rate into the EBZ.

Measuring calories

Table 7–4 will help you assess the calorie benefits of the time you spend doing model program 3. Use this Table to guide and measure your progress toward an energy expenditure of 200 to 350 calories each session. Walking and jogging for thirty minutes, covering about one and a half to two and a half miles, will cause a typical exerciser to burn about 200 to 350 calories each exercise session, totaling about 600 to 1,050 calories a week with three workouts a week. For a person with low to moderate CRE levels, that calorie cost—if expended by working within the EBZ—is enough to guarantee progress in improving CRE fitness.

Model program 4: jogging/running

Purpose: To develop and maintain a high level of cardiorespiratory fitness, a lean body, and muscular endurance.

Intensity. The key is to keep within your EBZ. Most people who sustain a continuous jog/run program will find that they can stay within their EBZ at a rate of speed between 5.5 and 7.5 miles per hour. Find out for yourself what intensity keeps you in your EBZ.

Duration. Start by jogging steadily for fifteen minutes. Gradually increase your jog/run session to a regular thirty to sixty minutes (or about two and a half to seven miles).

Frequency. Exercise every other day. Exercise more frequently—but alternate with other activities (see below)—if your purpose includes achieving a lean body.

Calorie cost. Use about 300 to 750 calories in each session. (See Table 7–7.)

Progesssion. If you chose model program 4, you probably already have moderate to high CRE. To improve CRE further, increase your distance or both pace and distance to burn additional calories. But make these adjustments only if you need to get your heart rate into the EBZ.

At the beginning

When you start this program, you already can jog comfortably for fifteen minutes without any muscular discomfort. But with this program you will be gradually increasing the time you spend jogging, and doing it in a way that prevents muscle and joint problems. Be consistent about your warm-up stretching. Do not make the commitment to this model program if you're likely to skimp on time for warm-up and cool-down.

If one of your purposes in exercising is to achieve a lean body, and if your exercise time is limited, model program 4 can make an effective contribution. The greater number of calories you burn per minute (see Table 7–7) makes this regimen less time-consuming for altering body composition and losing weight than the three previous programs in the walking/jogging/running series.

Even if you have ample time for daily exercise you still may wish to use model program 4. If your purpose is to lose weight or change body composition, do not use the model every day. Instead, on alternate days do long-distance walking (see model program 2) or some other high-calorie activity such as swimming or bicycling. Increasing frequency by using these supplemental activities will place less stress on the weight-bearing parts of the lower body than a daily regimen of jogging/running.

M.A., a Seattle pediatrician, told Consumers Union he began jogging at age thirty, when he weighed 200 pounds—too much, he thought, for his 6-foot frame. After about two weeks of jogging, M.A. built up to one mile. After two months, he was doing two miles. After six months, he could jog five miles at about 9 to 10 minutes per mile. By the end of a year he was jogging the five miles at about 7:30 minutes per mile, and found he had to force himself to slow down. M.A. warns beginners to resist the temptation to run too fast: "The goal is either distance or time, not speed. Speed is the enemy."

Table 7–7

Determining Calorie Cost Using Model Program 4

This Table gives the approximate calorie costs of a jogging/running program from 15 to 60 minutes for distances from 1.25 to 8 miles at varying rates of speed on a level terrain. (For a slower pace, refer to Table 7–4.) To use the Table, find on the horizontal line the approximate length of time you jog/run. Then locate on the vertical column the approximate distance you cover. The figure at the intersection represents an estimate of the calories used per pound of body weight. Multiply this figure by your own body weight to get the total number of calories used. For example, assuming you weigh 135 pounds and jog 3 miles in 30 minutes, you would burn 325 calories: 2.41 (calories per pound, from Table) × 135 (weight) = 325 calories.

Distance (in miles)	Time (in minutes)									
	15	20	25	30	35	40	45	50	55	60
1.25	.90									
1.50	1.20									
1.75	1.39									
2.00	1.57	1.61								
2.25	1.75	1.79								
2.50	1.93	1.97	2.01							
2.75		2.15	2.19	2.23						
3.00		2.33	2.37	2.41						
3.25		2.51	2.55	2.59	2.63					
3.50			2.73	2.77	2.81					
3.75			2.91	2.95	2.99	3.03				
4.00			3.09	3.13	3.17	3.21				
4.25				3.31	3.35	3.39	3.43			
4.50				3.49	3.53	3.57	3.61			
4.75					3.72	3.75	3.79	3.83		
5.00					3.90	3.94	3.98	4.01		
5.25					4.08	4.12	4.16	4.20	4.23	
5.50						4.30	4.34	4.38	4.42	4.46
5.75						4.48	4.52	4.56	4.60	4.64
6.00							4.70	4.74	4.78	4.82
6.25							4.88	4.92	4.96	5.00
6.50								5.10	5.14	5.18
6.75								5.28	5.32	5.36
7.00									5.50	5.54
7.25									5.68	5.72
7.50									5.86	5.90
7.75										6.08
8.00										6.27

During his year of jogging, M.A. reported he lost about twelve pounds "despite eating everything and anything I want." Describing himself as "an addicted runner," M.A. said his "mental condition is probably even greater than my physical."

As you progress

With a conditioning and maintenance program, it sometimes becomes necessary to forestall boredom. You can ease the monotony of the routine by varying the route, the intensity, and the duration. You may want to alternate short runs with long ones. If you run for sixty minutes one day, try running for thirty minutes for your next exercise session. Or try doing sets that alternate hard and easy intervals—even walking, if you feel like it. You could also try a road race now and then, but be careful not to do too much too soon.

Measuring calories

Table 7–7 will help you assess the calorie benefits of time spent doing model program 4. Use the Table to guide and measure your progress toward burning the recommended 300 to 750 calories in each session.

Model program 5: running (racing)

Purpose: To train for road races as a way of maintaining a high level of cardiorespiratory fitness, a lean body, and muscular endurance.

Intensity. Once again, it is important to stay within your EBZ. In a road race, you should aim to complete the distance at a pace roughly equal to the one you use in your regular workouts. If you find a need to increase your work load, observe the 10 percent rule: no more than a 10 percent increase in intensity or duration each week.

Duration. Your workouts should range from thirty to sixty minutes of running within your EBZ. For your first race, find a "fun run"* that covers no more than three to five miles. Only after several of these should you try races over longer distances.

Frequency. Keep your participation in road racing to less than once a month. Frequency of workouts should be every other day. If you want to exercise more often, add other activities (see model program 4) on alternate days.

Calorie cost. Use about 300 to 750 calories in each session.

Progression. Racing is not for everyone. But if you're a runner who enjoys competition and if you have the self-discipline to stick with a sensible rate of progress, road racing (or fun runs) can motivate you to achieve high levels of CRE. Training for road racing can be kept interesting and exciting: Add diversity to your sessions by using different training techniques (see pages 126–127).

---

*"Fun runs" are local runs over measured distances. The emphasis is on one's personal accomplishment rather than on competition against others.

A sample four-week program to train you for a first race of up to 5 miles is shown in Table 7–8.

Table 7–8

Training Program for 5-Mile Road Race

The Table below outlines a sample four-week program for preparing for a first road race of five miles or less. It uses long slow distance (LSD), interval training, and *fartlek* (see pages 126–127) to illustrate how these techniques can be combined effectively. Of course, a regimen can be based on just one of the three, but the combination provides a more diversified and perhaps more interesting approach to training.* The regimen calls for stretching exercises on most alternate days. See stretching model program.

Week I

Day 1   Run 30 to 60 minutes of LSD at a pace within your EBZ.
Day 2   Do stretching exercises.
Day 3   Do 30 to 60 minutes of *fartlek* on varied terrain at varied pace. Try to maintain your heart rate in your EBZ, but don't worry if your running segments bring your heart rate above your EBZ now and then. If done for an extended period, however, this can limit the duration of the session.
Day 4   Do stretching exercises.
Day 5   Run 30 to 60 minutes of LSD at a pace in the low to midrange of your EBZ.
Day 6   Do interval training. Run 440 yards at your time-goal pace (see Table 7–9, below), then walk 30 to 90 seconds. Repeat the set 16 times. The length of the walk interval depends on how long it takes to bring your heart rate below your EBZ.
Day 7   Do stretching exercises.

Week II

Day 1   Run 30 to 60 minutes of LSD at a pace in the low to midrange of your EBZ.
Day 2   Do stretching exercises.
Day 3   Do 30 to 60 minutes of *fartlek*.
Day 4   Do stretching exercises.
Day 5   Run 30 to 60 minutes of LSD within your EBZ.
Day 6   Do interval training. Run 880 yards at your time-goal pace, then walk 60 to 90 seconds. Repeat the set 10 times.
Day 7   Do stretching exercises.

Week III

Day 1   Run 30 to 60 minutes of LSD at a pace within your EBZ.

---

*Interval training complicates calorie calculations. A record of total time and distance covered will give you only an indication of calories used. To get an idea of calorie cost, see Table 7–7.

Day 2   Do stretching exercises.
Day 3   Do 30 to 60 minutes of *fartlek.*
Day 4   Do stretching exercises.
Day 5   Run 30 to 60 minutes of LSD within your EBZ.
Day 6   Do interval training. Run 1 mile at your time-goal pace, then walk 220 yards, and jog 220 yards at a slow pace. Repeat the set 5 times.
Day 7   Do stretching exercises.

Week IV (race week)

Day 1   Run 30 to 60 minutes of LSD at a pace within your EBZ.
Day 2   Do stretching exercises.
Day 3   Do interval training. Run 440 yards at your time-goal pace, then jog 220 yards at a slow pace. Repeat the set 16 times.
Day 4   Do stretching exercises.
Day 5   Run 30 minutes of LSD at a pace within your EBZ.
Day 6   Do stretching exercises.
Day 7   Run 5-mile race.

At the beginning

Try to finish your first race while running at your usual workout pace. You may finish at the back of the pack, but that's fine if that's where your current fitness level places you. While racing, don't be seduced by the excitement of competition. The surge of the crowd at the start, the tendency to set a fast pace, the adrenaline flowing freely, and sometimes an overwhelming desire to be a winner can trap you into running faster than you need to in order to stay within your EBZ. You're participating in regularly scheduled road races to help you stick with a regimen that will keep your CRE levels high and your body lean, but not necessarily to win the races.

By the time most runners take part in road races, they can tell when they're within their EBZ without having to take their pulse constantly. Should you need to check your EBZ, find another runner to chat with during the race, and rely on the talk test to adjust your pace.

Space your races to less than one a month; give yourself ample time to recover. And listen to your body. Each person is different in this regard. If you sense that you don't feel right in a race, avoid the tendency to "gut" it out. It's no disgrace to stop or slow down. If you feel like it, walk up a hill or stop for a drink of water. Hot days in particular can be a problem. (See Chapter 12 for more about running in hot weather.)

P.L., a fifty-year-old schoolteacher from Portage, Indiana, described for Consumers Union the culmination of his yearlong progression from jogging to regular road racing. "Last Saturday I entered a 5-kilometer (3.1-mile) race. I came in second in my age group [over 50] with a time of 26:16. The winning time was run by a doctor—19:45. This was only the third race I had entered, and I finished second. What more motivation does a young man of fifty need?" During his years of jogging/running,

125

P.L. reports losing fifteen pounds, and his double chin and pot belly "are almost gone."

As you progress

The key is slow steady progress: Increase mileage and pace by no more than 10 percent a week. You may not win the races you enter, but you're more likely to be free of injuries. At your own rate of progress, your satisfaction will come from setting occasional personal records—improving your time, adding to your distance, or moving up in the order of finish.

For many runners, a marathon seems the ultimate achievement. If you want to run in a marathon, be sure to progress slowly. Only after you have gradually and systematically worked up to longer distances should you set yourself such a challenge.

Marathoners and beginning road racers alike benefit from many of the same training techniques. When training for a race, there are several ways to add variety to your regimen.

Long slow distance (LSD). This technique—running at a comfortable level within the EBZ for prolonged durations—is the foundation of your running program. LSD should also be the mainstay of your preparation for racing. Increase the length of your runs; if you stay within your EBZ, your CRE will improve and your intensity will automatically increase without conscious effort. Forget about dramatic efforts to make your super-racer fantasies come true: They may lead to injuries and spoil a good fitness program. If on occasion you want to run faster, try interval training or *fartlek* (see below).

Interval training. By scheduling a resting interval alternately with a running interval—each combination is one set—interval training lets you extend a workout over a longer time. This technique delays the onset of fatigue. Suppose you want to prepare for a five-mile race that you hope to run in forty minutes—a pace of 8 minutes per mile. You would then plan to run 10 or more half-mile intervals at your pace or better (see Table 7–8). For resting intervals, you would walk or jog for up to ninety seconds or until your EBZ dips below minimum threshold levels.

With interval training, you can vary the distance and pace of the running period and the number of sets you do. The number and length of your resting intervals affects the intensity of the workout, as does the pace at which you run. Keep your workout interval below the upper level of your EBZ. Although there's no harm in a well-conditioned runner exceeding the EBZ now and then, overdoing it results in fatigue and limits the duration of the workout. See Table 7–9 for suggestions on pace.

Fartlek is Swedish for "play of speed." It's a training technique you can use when you want a change of pace from LSD. Just as LSD is steady and sensible, *fartlek* is freewheeling and unpredictable. With this technique, you can run as fast or slow as you like for as long or short a period as you choose, mixing sprints and walking in a long, unplanned, untimed, cross-country run in the woods, on beaches, up and down hills, or in any setting that provides a pleasant change of pace. The short bursts of speed can be exhilarating after a period on LSD training and the lack of structure can be welcome after interval training.

Table 7–9

Walking/Jogging/Running Pace Chart

This Table provides approximate times for distances from 110 yards to 5 miles and for rates of speed from 3 to 11 miles per hour. Use this Table to set your time-goals for interval training.

Activity	Miles per hour	Distances (in hours:minutes:seconds)					
		5 miles	1 mile	880 yds. (½ mile)	440 yds. (¼ mile)	220 yds.	110 yds.
Walking							
Moderate	3.0	1:40:00	20:00	10:00	5:00	2:30	1:15
	3.75	1:20:00	16:00	8:00	4:00	2:00	1:00
Fast	4.5	1:07:45	13:33	6:46	3:23	1:41	:50
Jogging							
Slow	5.0	60:00	12:00	6:00	3:00	1:30	:45
	5.5	55:00	11:00	5:30	2:45	1:23	:41
Moderate	6.0	50:00	10:00	5:00	2:30	1:15	:37
	6.7	45:00	9:00	4:30	2:15	1:08	:34
Fast	7.0	42:55	8:35	4:18	2:09	1:04	:32
	7.5	40:00	8:00	4:00	2:00	1:00	:30
Running							
Slow	8.6	35:00	7:00	3:30	1:45	:53	:26
Moderate	9.0	33:20	6:40	3:20	1:40	:50	:25
Fast	10.0	30:00	6:00	3:00	1:30	:45	:22
	11.0	27:30	5:30	2:45	1:23	:41	:20

Interval circuit training

Interval circuit training is a series of exercises, performed in sequence, and using several pieces of equipment (see Equipment, below). This model program of nine exercises provides a workout for all major muscle groups and has the potential of improving CRE, muscular strength, and muscular endurance. With this program, you can burn about 10 calories per minute.

In interval circuit training, each exercise should be performed at your maximum effort for thirty seconds, followed by fifteen seconds in which you record the number of repetitions performed and prepare for the next exercise. (See Table 7–10 for a sample progress chart.)

Terminology

To use interval circuit training, you have to learn the language—some of which may be new to you.

Circuit training. A system of organizing a series of exercises arranged for consecutive performance. In this program, nine exercises is one circuit.

Repetitions. The number of times you perform an exercise.

Exercise interval. The time in which you perform an exercise at your maximum effort. For this program, thirty seconds is the exercise interval.

Rest interval. The time following the performance of an exercise, used to record the number of repetitions completed and to prepare for the next exercise. For this program, fifteen seconds is the rest interval.

Interval circuit training program

Purpose. To develop and maintain all fitness components, primarily CRE and muscular endurance.

Equipment. One barbell, one swingbell (dumbbell bar with plates clamped in the center of the bar), slant board, bench or chair, jump rope, wand (broomsticklike length of wood doweling), cassette and player (or large-faced clock with sweep-second hand).

Intensity. Because this model program is designed for muscular endurance, you'll exercise against low resistance with many repetitions. Because you exercise at high intensity (performing at maximum effort, i.e., as many repetitions as you can within a limited time), there is a fifteen-second rest interval between the performance of each exercise. The exercises are arranged so that the same muscle groups are not used in successive exercises, thus avoiding overtiring them.

Heart rates have been recorded at high levels during the performance of this model program. So monitor your pulse periodically and raise or lower the intensity (number of repetitions) to keep your heart rate within your exercise benefit zone (see pages 62–66).

Duration. Do three trips around the circuit, which should take about twenty minutes. That's enough to influence CRE. One or two circuits take

Table 7–10

Log for Interval Circuit Training Program

In this sample progress chart for interval circuit training, the first column shows the exercises in the order they should be performed. The figures in the second column (1, 2, 3) represent the first, second, and third times around the circuit. In the other columns, enter the number of repetitions performed for the exercises each time you make your way around the circuit. As a guide, we have filled in the number of repetitions for what could be one day in each of your first three weeks on the model program. First week: once around the circuit on three alternate days. Second week: two consecutive turns around the circuit on three alternate days. Third week and weeks following: three consecutive turns around the circuit on three alternate days. When you want to add weight (+ wt.) to your equipment, you can record it as shown below.

Exercise		1st week	2nd week	3rd week	
1. Bent rowing	1. 2. 3.	20	20 21	20 + wt. 16 18	
2. Sit-up	1. 2. 3.	18	19 17	18 16 17	
3. Clean and press	1. 2. 3.	17	17 18	18 16 18	
4. Curl	1. 2. 3.	25	26 + wt. 26	24 25 24	
5. Twister	1. 2. 3.	45	50 48	45 40 40	
6. Forward raise	1. 2. 3.	18	20 19	19 16 18	
7. Step-up	1. 2. 3.	20	19 20	19 17 19	
8. Push-up	1. 2. 3.	13	12 10	14 12 12	
9. Rope skipping	1. 2. 3.	25	35 31	35 30 35	

129

less time, and can be effective in developing muscular endurance. But fewer than three circuits would be of limited significance in improving CRE.

Frequency. Exercise three days per week.

At the beginning

At a local fitness center or store that carries weight training equipment, experiment with a barbell until you find a weight you can use for at least 15 repetitions without strain.

After you have assembled all your equipment, set it up in your workout area so you can perform each exercise in the thirty seconds allowed. Read the instructions carefully on how to perform the exercises.

Always warm up. Do the stretching model program before you start your exercise period. To prevent excessive soreness, limit yourself to just one full circuit for the first three exercise periods. Go on to two full circuits for the next three exercise periods. From then on, each exercise period should consist of three complete circuits. A cassette can help you control your time around the circuit. Using a stopwatch, record your own voice saying: "Ready, begin. . . . Record and change," etc., allowing thirty seconds for the exercise interval followed by fifteen seconds for the rest interval.

Exercises for interval circuit training program

Refer to the Glossary of Exercises for instructions on how to perform most of the exercises in this model program. For best results, do the exercises in the numerical sequence below. It's important to perform at your maximum effort for the thirty-second exercise interval (followed by the fifteen-second rest interval in which to record and change). Doing the circuit as a whole will improve CRE. The body parts affected by the exercises are noted, as well as which exercises are especially useful for CRE.

---

1. Bent rowing: Barbell
(See Glossary 3B)

Upper back, arms

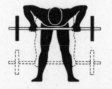

130

2. Sit-up: Slant board
(See Glossary 24E)

Abdominals

3. Clean and press: Barbell
(See Glossary 4B)

Full body

4. Curl: Barbell
(See Glossary 7B)

Biceps, forearms

5. Twister: Wand
(See Glossary 3E)

Hamstrings, trunk

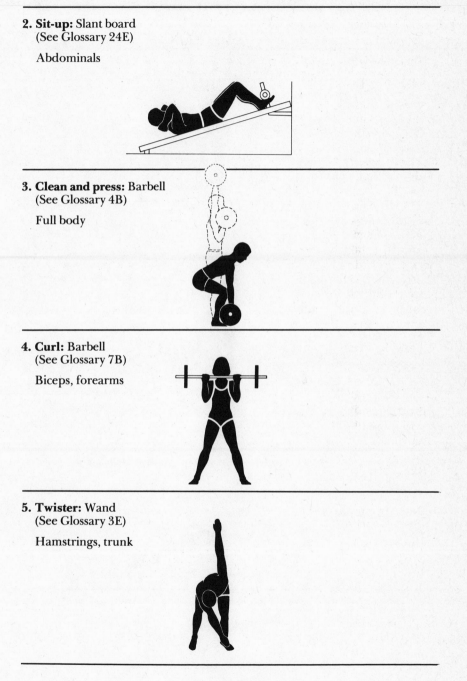

6. Forward raise: Dumbbells
(See Glossary 2D)

Shoulders, upper back

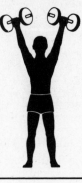

7. Step-up: Bench or chair
(See Glossary 23E)

Thighs, hips, CRE

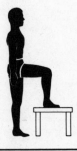

8. Push-up
(See Glossary 25E)

Chest, triceps, upper back

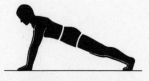

9. Rope skipping: Rope
(See rope skipping model program)

CRE, legs

Calisthenic circuit training

Calisthenics (from the Greek, meaning beautiful strength) is a series of rhythmic exercises, usually performed without apparatus, to develop muscular strength, muscular endurance, and flexibility. Because you need little or no equipment, calisthenics allows you to perform your exercises at home or while traveling. As commonly practiced, such exercises are not a well-rounded fitness program. Using the model program based on *circuit training,* however, can increase the value of calisthenics for fitness. This model program consists of twelve exercises.

Terminology

Here are the terms you'll need to know in doing this model program.

Circuit training. A system of organizing a series of exercises arranged for consecutive performance. Exercises for different muscle groups follow each other, which helps delay the onset of fatigue. When all twelve exercises in this model program have been performed, one circuit is completed. Three trips around the circuit are required for this model program. Because you're striving for a *target time* (see below), you need to record your time for completing the three trips around the circuit. At first, of course, it takes a longer time to complete the circuit, but as you improve in fitness, you will improve your time (you'll need less rest and your pace will quicken).

Repetitions. The number of times you perform an exercise.

Target time. For this model program, twenty minutes is the target time—the time within which you hope to complete three circuits. When you hit your target, increase the number of repetitions of each exercise.

Work description. At first, your work description is one-half of your maximum effort. For example, if you can do 16 push-ups in one minute (your maximum effort), your work description is 8 push-ups in one minute. Performing your exercises at one-half of your maximum effort for three trips around the circuit provides progressive overload. (With a maximum effort of 16 push-ups and a work description of 8 push-ups, you would do 8 push-ups for each of three trips around the circuit for a total of 24 push-ups—8 more than your maximum effort of 16—thus providing progressive overload.) Your work description will increase as you become more fit.

Calisthenic circuit training program

Purpose. To develop and maintain CRE, muscular strength, muscular endurance, and flexibility of the major joints.

Equipment. This model program requires no special equipment. But a stopwatch would be useful to record time.

Intensity. Determine intensity by testing yourself on each exercise in the circuit to find out how many times you can perform the exercises in the given time. (Testing yourself over a two-day period will reduce the chance of muscle soreness.) You increase intensity by working faster and by increasing repetitions when the twenty-minute target time is achieved. When you can complete three circuits in the target time, increase the repetitions for each exercise by one-fourth of your work description. For example, if your work description is 8 push-ups (one-half of your maximum effort), increase your repetitions to 10 push-ups. Even with this one-fourth increase in repetitions, you should eventually perform the three circuits in the twenty-minute target time. After you have achieved the twenty-minute target time, increase your work description by one-fourth.

Be sure to monitor your pulse rate during the calisthenic circuit so your heart rate stays within your exercise benefit zone (see pages 62–66). If your heart rate is high, slow your pace.

Duration. Exercise for the length of time it takes you to do three complete circuits. Your aim is to complete three circuits in the target time of twenty minutes, but as you work toward target time, expect to take longer than twenty minutes.

Frequency. Exercise a minimum of three days per week.

At the beginning

Although a warm-up is built into the calisthenic circuit training model program, you should still warm up before you begin each workout (see stretching model program). To establish your work description, test yourself (over two days) to determine how much effort you have to use in order to complete each of the twelve exercises within the time limit. After you have arrived at your work description for each exercise, use it to perform one full circuit for the first three exercise periods. Go on to two full circuits for the next three exercise periods. From then on, each exercise period should consist of three complete circuits. Keep a note pad handy to jot down the date and the time it takes to complete three full circuits. When you can finish three circuits in the target time of twenty minutes, you're ready to increase the repetitions of each exercise and thus increase your work description.

Exercises for calisthenic circuit training program

Refer to the Glossary of Exercises for instructions on how to perform most of the exercises in this model program. For best results, do the exercises in the numerical sequence below. Count the number of times you can complete each exercise in the time limit given, and enter that number as your maximum effort. One-half of this is your work description.

When performing the circuit, complete your work description for each exercise as rapidly as possible. When you can do three trips around the circuit in twenty minutes, increase your work description. Doing the circuit as a whole will improve CRE. The body parts affected by the exercises are noted for each part of the circuit, as well as which exercises are especially useful for CRE.

---

1. Arm circles: Time limit, 30 sec.
(See Glossary 2E)

Shoulders

Maximum effort_____
Work description_____.

---

2. Jumping jack: Time limit, 1 min.
(See Glossary 6E)

CRE, legs

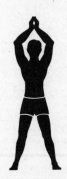

Maximum effort_____
Work description_____.

---

3. Push-up: Time limit, 1 min.
(See Glossary 25E)

Chest, triceps, upper back

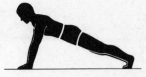

Maximum effort_____
Work description_____.

---

4. Parallel squat: Time limit, 1 min.
(See Glossary 9E)

Quadriceps, hips

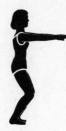

Maximum effort_____
Work description_____.

5. Sit-up: Time limit, 1 min.
(See Glossary 24E)

Abdominals

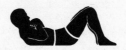

Maximum effort_____
Work description_____.

6. Side leg raise: Time limit, 1 min.
(See Glossary 16E)

Thighs, hips

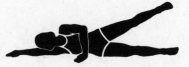

Maximum effort_____
Work description_____.

7. Knee-to-chest: Time limit, 1 min.
(See Glossary 14E)

Abdominals, hips, lower back

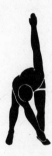

Maximum effort_____
Work description_____.

---

8. Alternate toe touch: Time limit,
1 min.
(See Glossary 4E)

Hamstrings, trunk

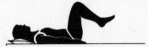

Maximum effort_____
Work description_____.

---

9. Squat thrust: Time limit, 1 min.
(See Glossary 11E)

Trunk, hips, thighs, arms

Maximum effort_____
Work description_____.

---

10. Shoulder bridge: Time limit,
1 min.
(See Glossary 19E)

Lower back

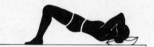

Maximum effort_____
Work description_____.

11. Side bend: Time limit, 1 min.
(See Glossary 5E)

Trunk

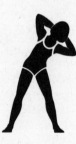

Maximum effort_____
Work description_____.

12. Run in place: Time limit, 3 min.

CRE, legs

Maximum effort
(number of steps)_____
Work description_____.

Stretching

Stretching develops the flexibility component of physical fitness, and should be included in the warm-up (before) and cool-down (after) for all fitness programs. It can also be a fitness program in itself.

Two stretching model programs are presented here: The first is a basic stretching program of ten exercises that include movements for most major joints and muscle groups. The second, an eleven-part program, is designed as a warm-up/cool-down for most activities, particularly for walking/jogging/running programs, bicycling, and rope skipping. By referring to the Glossary of Exercises you can, of course, design your own individualized program to meet your personal needs.

Terminology

Two terms are important in the stretching model programs.

Static stretching. To stretch as far as possible without any repetitive bouncing movements. This is the prescribed method of performing each stretching exercise.

Stretch reflex. A protective contraction of the muscle being stretched. It is the body's defense against overstretch and possible injury.

Basic stretching program

Purpose. To develop and maintain flexibility of the major joints of the body.

Intensity and duration. The intensity and duration for each of the exercises can best be explained in two phases.

1. The adjustment phase. Using static stretching, let muscles and other connective tissue gradually get used to the position. By moving slowly and easily into the stretching position, you will avoid the stretch reflex. Allow your body to relax and enjoy the melting away of that tight feeling. Hold the position for ten seconds. As you progress, your body adjusts to the stretching position, and you can gradually increase the time up to thirty seconds. There should be no exertion involved in the adjustment phase.

2. The development phase. Repeat the exercise, but now stretch a bit farther. Relax and focus on the pleasurable sensation as your muscles stretch to their limits without pain. Hold the position for fifteen seconds. As you progress, your body becomes accustomed to the stretching position and you can gradually increase the time up to sixty seconds.

Frequency. To be most effective, the basic stretching program—which consists of ten exercises involving the major joints and muscle groups—should be done daily.

At the beginning

Allow your body to move gently and gradually into the stretch position. Stretch slowly and gradually—avoid bouncing. Don't attempt to set records by forcing the stretch to the point of pain.

For the first four or five workouts, allow yourself to become familiar and comfortable with each movement and position. You will get optimal benefit only if you relax and enjoy stretching, whether you use it as a basic stretching program or as warm-up/cool-down.

Exercises for basic stretching program

Refer to the Glossary of Exercises for instructions on how to perform these exercises. For best results, do the exercises in the numerical sequence below. The body parts affected by the exercises are noted for each part of the stretching program.

1. Shoulder blade scratch
(See Glossary 18F)

Shoulders, arms

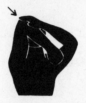

2. Towel stretch
(See Glossary 20F)

Triceps, shoulders, upper back

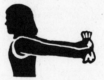

3. Alternate knee-to-chest
(See Glossary 5F)

Lower back

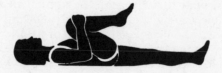

4. Double knee-to-chest
(See Glossary 6F)

Lower back

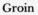

5. Sole stretch
(See Glossary 16F)

Groin

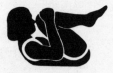

6. Seated toe touch no. 2
(See Glossary 4F)

Hamstrings

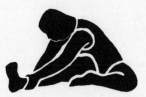

7. Seated foot-over-knee twist
(See Glossary 12F)

Hips

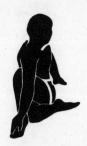

141

8. Prone knee flexion
(See Glossary 10F)

Quadriceps

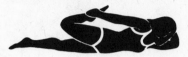

9. Wall lean
(See Glossary 14F)

Lower legs

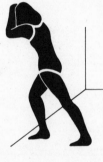

10. Stride stretch
(See Glossary 13F)

Hips, hamstrings

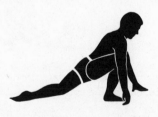

Warm-up/cool-down

Do the following exercises before and after most activities —particularly walking/jogging/running programs, bicycling, and rope skipping— to achieve and maintain flexibility. These exercises are done just once, as in the basic stretching program, except for the leg cross-overs and the sit-up, which should be done for 5 to 20 repetitions each.

Exercises for warm-up/cool-down

Refer to the Glossary of Exercises for instructions on how to perform these exercises. For best results, do the exercises in the numerical sequence below. The body parts affected by the exercises are noted for each part of the warm-up/cool-down program.

---

1. Alternate knee-to-chest
(See Glossary 5F)

Lower back

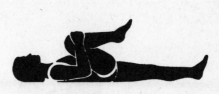

---

2. Leg cross-overs
(See Glossary 15E)

Hips, back

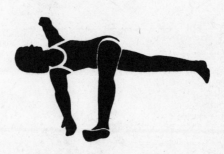

---

3. Double knee-to-chest
(See Glossary 6F)

Lower back

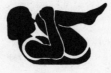

---

4. Sole stretch
(See Glossary 16F)

Groin

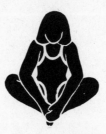

5. Seated toe touch no. 2
(See Glossary 4F)

Hamstrings

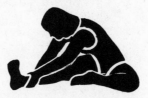

6. Sit-up
(See Glossary 24E)

Abdominals

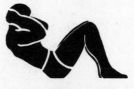

7. Seated foot-over-knee twist
(See Glossary 12F)

Hips

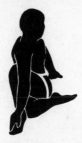

8. Back over
(See Glossary 7F)

Back, hamstrings

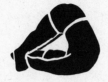

9. Prone knee flexion
(See Glossary 10F)

Quadriceps

10. Wall lean
(See Glossary 14F)

Lower legs

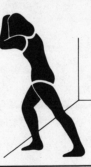

11. Standing toe touch
(See Glossary 1F)

Hamstrings

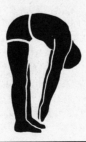

Bicycling

Bicycling (or "cycling") can be fun, be socially rewarding, and pay large dividends in physical fitness. It is a high calorie-per-minute activity that promotes changes in body composition and weight control. Fifteen minutes or longer of cycling at a speed fast enough to bring your heart rate into your exercise benefit zone (EBZ, see pages 62–66) is an excellent exercise for developing a high level of CRE. Also, cycling promotes muscular endurance and muscular strength, and improves flexibility of selected muscles of the legs and hips.

For many, cycling is a pleasant and economical alternative to the automobile and a convenient way to improve physical fitness. The advent of 10-speed bikes and their capacity to make uphill pedaling easy has popularized bikes for shopping, going to school, to work, and for errands. The growing number of bicycle paths and lanes in many communities has also led to more recreational cycling.

Many cyclists—after a time—join cycling groups on day, weekend, or vacation outings, which can cover hundreds of miles during a tour. (Bicycle racing, however, is a demanding sport that requires a high level of skill and fitness.)

Bicycling program

Purpose. To develop and maintain all five fitness components by cycling for at least fifteen consecutive minutes with your heart rate within your EBZ.

Equipment. Cycling has its own special array of equipment—including headgear, lighting, safety pennants, and special shoes. But it's the bike itself that requires the largest outlay, ranging from about $100 to as much as $1,000. Avoid a costly investment until you're sure you'll use your bike regularly. Consider renting or borrowing a bike while you investigate what the marketplace has to offer. Don't be influenced by the latest fad or a bike's appearance. The type you buy should be geared to your intended use of the bike. Most cyclists who are interested primarily in fitness are best served by a sturdy 10-speed.

When choosing clothing for bike riding, avoid restrictive or binding garments. But don't wear loose-fitting pants or long skirts that can be caught in the chain. While clothing worn on the upper body should be comfortable and loose, it should not be so loose as to catch the wind and slow you down. Whether you should use headgear is a question often raised. Some exercisers find a helmet uncomfortable, especially in warm weather. If you intend to ride in heavily trafficked areas, however, you should always use headgear.

Intensity, duration, and frequency. If you've been inactive for a long time, it may be wise to begin a cycling program at a heart rate that is 10 to 20 percent lower than your EBZ. If your heart rate is too high or if you feel uncomfortable, slow down or stop for a brief rest period (see At the beginning, below). Once you feel at home on your bike, try a mile at a comfortable speed. Then stop and check your heart rate response by taking your pulse. Don't be concerned if it still falls below your EBZ. After all, it may require several outings to get the muscles and joints of your legs and hips adjusted to this new activity. You should be able to increase your speed gradually, until you can cycle at 12 to 15 miles per hour, a speed fast enough to bring most new cyclists' heart rate into their EBZ. Cycling for at least fifteen minutes three times per week at this speed will lead to improvement in CRE.

When cycling you burn calories, and the more calories you burn the more effective your exercise program. Review Table 7–11 to determine the number of calories that you burn at each outing. You can increase the number of calories burned by cycling faster or for a longer duration. If you can spare the time, it's better to increase distance than to add speed. Don't push too hard. Let your body adapt: Allow your pulse rate to be your guide. More highly fit individuals may need to ride at faster than 13 to 15 miles per hour to achieve heart rates within their EBZ.

Interval training is also effective with cycling. Simply increase your speed for periods of four to eight minutes or for specific distances, one to two miles, say. Then coast for two or three minutes. Repeat the speed interval followed by the slow interval for a total of twenty to sixty minutes, depending on your level of fitness. The slow cycling will allow your heart rate to drop enough to recover in preparation for the next speed interval without a loss in exercise benefits. Cycling over hilly terrain is also a form of interval training: Pedaling uphill is the exercise interval, and coasting downhill is the rest interval.

At the beginning

Bike riding requires a number of precise skills that practice makes automatic. If you have biked in the past, you will shake off that rusty feeling after a few exploratory trips. If you have never ridden, investigate the possibility of a course at a nearby college, "Y," etc. (Many courses are not just for the neophyte. They help to develop braking, shifting, and emergency skills and teach ways of caring for and repairing your bike.) Until you become a skilled cyclist, select routes with the fewest hazards and avoid heavy automobile traffic.

Begin each outing with a ten-minute warm-up. (See warm-up/cool-down in stretching model program.) Pay particular attention to stretching the hamstrings because cycling tends to tighten them. Also, do not neglect stretching exercises for the back and neck muscles.

Safety tips

The National Injury Information Clearinghouse (a federal agency) classifies bicycle riding as the nation's most dangerous sport. Many of the

147

injuries are the result of the cyclist's carelessness. Fred Delong, in his book *Delong's Guide to Bicycles & Bicycling,* suggests that cyclists practice "preventive cycling." The following list is adapted from Delong's recommendations.

■ Keep on the correct side of the road. Bicycling against traffic is usually illegal and always dangerous.

■ Obey all traffic signs and signals.

Table 7–11

Determining Calorie Cost for Bicycling

This Table gives the approximate calorie costs per pound of body weight of cycling from 5 to 60 minutes for distances of .50 mile up to 15 miles on a level terrain. To use the Table, find on the horizontal line the time most closely approximating the number of minutes you cycle. Next, locate on the vertical column the approximate distance in miles you cover. The figure at the intersection represents an estimate of the calories used per minute per pound of body weight. Multiply this figure by your own body weight. Then multiply the product of these two figures by the number of minutes you cycle to get the total number of calories burned. For example, assuming you weigh 154 pounds and cycle 3 miles in 20 minutes, you would burn 130 calories: 154 × .042 (calories per pound, from Table) = 6.5 × 20 (minutes) = 130 calories burned.

Distance (in miles)	Time (in minutes)											
	5	10	15	20	25	30	35	40	45	50	55	60
.50	.032											
1.00	.062	.032										
1.50		.042	.032									
2.00		.062	.039	.032								
3.00			.062	.042	.036	.032						
4.00				.062	.044	.039	.035	.032				
5.00				.097	.062	.045	.041	.037	.035	.032		
6.00					.088	.062	.047	.042	.039	.036	.034	.032
7.00						.081	.062	.049	.043	.040	.038	.036
8.00							.078	.062	.050	.044	.041	.039
9.00								.076	.062	.051	.045	.042
10.00								.097	.074	.062	.051	.045
11.00									.093	.073	.062	.052
12.00										.088	.072	.062
13.00											.084	.071
14.00												.081
15.00												.097

■ On public roads, ride in a single file, except in low-traffic areas (if the law permits). Ride in a straight line; don't swerve or weave in traffic.

■ Be alert; anticipate movements of other traffic and pedestrians. Listen for approaching traffic that is out of your line of vision.

■ Slow down at street crossings. Check both ways before crossing.

■ Use hand signals—the same as for automobile drivers—if you intend to stop or turn. Use audible signals to warn those in your path.

■ Maintain full control. Avoid anything that interferes with your vision. Don't jeopardize your ability to steer by carrying anything (including people) on the handlebars.

■ Maintain your bicycle in good shape with attachments securely tightened, and brakes, gears, saddle, wheels, and tires all in good condition.

■ See and be seen. Use a headlight at night; equip your bike with rear reflectors. Use side reflectors on pedals, front and rear. Wear light-colored clothing or use reflective tape at night and bright colors or fluorescent tape by day.

■ Be courteous to other road users. Anticipate the worst, and practice preventive cycling.

Common cycling ailments

Some cycling ailments are bothersome but easy to prevent. Others should be treated promptly to avoid having to discontinue cycling.

Saddle soreness. Saddle soreness is due to two conditions: pressure on the soft tissue of the genital area and on the buttocks that may cause pain, tingling, or numbness; and chafing caused by friction on the skin of the buttocks. These problems can be prevented or reduced by the following measures.

■ Use a comfortable saddle, one that is reasonably soft (or softened with padding or a leather softener). Adjust the saddle to a comfortable height. The height you select should allow your legs to almost reach full extension while pedaling. During long rides you may find it comfortable to periodically change the tilt of the saddle slightly. Frequently change the position of your body on the saddle. Also adjust the handlebars to change your body position.

■ Wear a pair of cycling pants or shorts padded by soft chamois sewn in the seat to act as a cushion and reduce friction. The liberal use of talcum powder or cornstarch can also help reduce friction. It may be wise to carry a supply if you go on a trip. Once irritation has formed, petroleum jelly can be useful (though messy). Consult a physician about skin infections.

Numb hands. Long trips may result in a numbness of the hands. You can try to prevent this by wearing well-padded gloves. You can also pad the handlebars with foam and periodically shift and alter the position of your hands on the handlebars.

Backache and neck strain. Beginning cyclists may suffer from backache and neck strain. These may be due to the stretching demands of cycling to which new cyclists are not accustomed. To prevent strains, do exercises designed to stretch the back and neck muscles during your warm-up. In time, the discomfort should disappear.

Rope skipping

Rope skipping can be an excellent fitness program. It's inexpensive, convenient, and an effective exercise for high levels of CRE and muscular endurance of the lower legs. It can also help with weight loss. And it's a fine rainy day alternative for outdoor CRE activities such as jogging or bicycling.

There are many ways to skip rope, but the most common techniques are jumping on one foot at a time or both feet together, with or without an added bounce. Select the technique that feels best to you. There isn't much difference in the difficulty or energy demands of the various techniques.

At first, you may be grateful to get over the rope in *any* manner. But after a while skipping rope could become boring if done for long periods of time within the confines of four walls. In time you'll be able to try a variety of approaches—alternating among single jumping on first one foot and then the other, both feet at the same time, crossing your arms over your head, and changing the direction of the rope from front swing to back swing. With a little imagination (and experimentation) you'll be able to create some variations of your own. You could also try skipping rope while watching television or listening to the radio. Some people find that music helps to keep a rhythm.

Rope skipping does little for acquiring and maintaining flexibility. It does develop some strength in the legs and forearms. Because of the muscular demands of rope skipping, it's especially important to warm up adequately. Do stretching exercises for the lower back, lower legs, and hamstrings. (See warm-up/cool-down in stretching model program.)

Terminology

Rope skipping is relatively simple, and so is the language you use.

Turns per minute. This refers to the number of times in one minute the rope passes under your feet.

Set. One set consists of a combination of an interval of rope skipping for a specific time followed by a rest interval for a specific time.

Rope skipping program

Purpose. To develop and maintain CRE and muscular endurance of the lower legs by skipping rope for fifteen minutes (including rest intervals) with your heart rate within your exercise benefit zone (EBZ, see pages 62–66).

Equipment. First, there is the rope. Use the correct length (long enough to reach from armpit to armpit, passing under both feet). It can be made of nylon, plastic, hemp, rubber, or leather. Store-bought ropes often come with handles or special grips with weights or ball bearings to use for recording the number of turns. You may find this useful, but start out with clothesline or a simple inexpensive jump rope until you're sure you will continue the exercise. (Jump ropes vary in price from $3 to $15.) Because rope skipping requires constant impact on the metatarsal bones (the ball of the foot), a good pair of jogging shoes may be helpful. In any case, wear comfortable supportive sneakers or running shoes. And a watch or clock can be useful to record time.

Intensity and duration. Rope skipping as a form of interval training uses sets of skipping intervals alternating with rest intervals, gradually increasing the skipping time at the expense of the rest time.

A good starting program for beginning rope skippers is to do one set of fifteen seconds of rope skipping followed by fifteen to thirty seconds of rest. Increase the number of sets gradually as your legs, arms, and CRE begin to make the necessary adjustments. (See Table 7–12 for a sample rope skipping program.) Periodically check your pulse rate so that your heart rate stays within your EBZ: Increase or slow down your turns per minute as needed.

It is important to remember to monitor your heart rate carefully. You may want to keep your heart rate 10 to 20 percent below your EBZ at the beginning. As your condition improves, you will be able to increase your skipping intervals and decrease your rest intervals. Eventually, you may be able to skip rope for fifteen minutes or longer without stopping—even though it is not necessary to do so. You can achieve high levels of CRE and muscular endurance on the interval skipping program. Continue to add skipping/resting sets until your total rope skipping intervals—not counting rest intervals—add up to fifteen minutes. As your CRE and muscular endurance improve, you may find you can increase the intensity (turns of the rope per minute) to keep your heart rate within your EBZ.

Frequency. Because of the constant impact on the feet, it's wise to limit rope skipping to every other day. Or you could alternate it with other forms of CRE exercise such as bicycling, walking, or swimming to limit any trauma to the feet.

At the beginning

How to skip rope can present a modest challenge to the novice. And even if you've been an active rope skipper in the past, you may find that now your legs and arms tire very quickly. Rope skipping is vigorous exercise and too demanding for most sedentary people without a gradual introduction. As with prospective joggers, inexperienced rope skippers should start out with a period of walking to begin the necessary muscular and CRE adjustment to rope skipping. The first step in a rope skipping program for beginners, therefore, should be completing model program 1: walking (starting).

Ease into rope skipping if you have limited skill. Start gradually, allowing muscles and CRE to adjust. Skip on firm but resilient surfaces.

Start by practicing the "rope twirl," by doubling the rope and placing

---

Table 7–12

Sample Rope Skipping Program

This Table gives calorie costs for eleven different rope skipping programs. The resting and skipping intervals shown are suggestions only. You can increase or decrease the intervals and the number of sets by one or two as necessary to keep within your EBZ. The approximate calories per pound are for skipping intervals at a rate of 70 turns per minute. (See Chapter 8 for information about calories burned while rope skipping at 80, 90, and 100 turns per minute.) To find the total calories burned, multiply your weight by the appropriate number of calories per pound. For example, if you skip rope for 3 minutes (first column) with 60-second rest intervals (second column) and you do 6 sets (third column), the total time skipping rope is 18 minutes and you would burn 1.3 calories per pound. If you weigh 154 pounds, you'd burn approximately 200 calories: 154 × 1.3 (calories per pound, from Table) = 200 calories burned.

Skipping interval (minutes: seconds)	Rest interval (minutes: seconds)	Number of sets	Total skipping time (in minutes)	Approximate calories used per pound
0:15	0:30	4–10	1–2.5	.07–.18
0:30	0:30	5–10	2.5–6	.18–.43
0:45	0:30	8–12	6–8	.43–.57
0:60	0:30	6–12	8–12	.57–.86
1:30	0:30	8–10	12–15	.86–1.1
2:00	0:60	8	16	1.2
3:00	0:60	6	18	1.3
6:00	1:30	3	18	1.3
9:00	1:30	2	18	1.3
12:00	2:00	2	24	1.7
15:00	0:00	1	15	1.1

both handles of the rope in one hand. Twirl the rope forward in a circular motion and every time the rope hits the floor, you jump. Practice the rope twirl with the rope in one hand for fifteen seconds, rest fifteen to thirty seconds, then begin the rope twirl again with the rope in the other hand. Once you've mastered the rope twirl, you're ready to start skipping rope. Begin slowly. Select a pace that is comfortable—60 turns per minute should be right for most beginners. As you become more proficient, you will be able to skip from 70 to more than 100 turns per minute.

Many activities designed to promote CRE consist of continued rhythmic activities within your EBZ for at least fifteen minutes. Rope skipping for fifteen uninterrupted minutes, however, presents more muscular stress than other CRE activities (jogging, for example). So it may not even be practical for people with limited muscular endurance or who have muscle and joint problems. What's more, it's difficult to skip rope for fifteen minutes at a rate of 50 to 60 turns per minute and still maintain a rhythm. At that rate, heart response for beginners may tend to go beyond the EBZ very quickly. The sample rope skipping program (Table 7–12) is designed to help you keep your heart rate within your EBZ by showing you how to use rest intervals.

Swimming

One of the best all-around exercises, swimming is a large-muscle, rhythmic activity that is self-paced. Like jogging and bicycling, it has excellent potential for bringing your heart rate into your exercise benefit zone (EBZ, see pages 62–66), and thus for developing a high level of CRE.

The most common swimming strokes are the crawl (freestyle), sidestroke, elementary backstroke, breaststroke, and arm-over-arm backstroke. Swimming, using any one or a combination of these strokes for fifteen consecutive minutes, develops muscular strength. Most strokes also encourage shoulder joint flexibility and high levels of muscular endurance. Some people find swimming helpful for changing body composition. It is because swimming develops all five fitness components that it is so highly rated as a well-rounded exercise.

Terminology

The language for this model program is familiar to most swimmers.
Lap. One width or one length of a pool, regardless of pool size.

Swimming program

Purpose. To develop and maintain all five fitness components by swimming fifteen consecutive minutes with your heart rate within your EBZ.

Equipment. Swimming goggles to protect your eyes from irritation in chlorinated pools.

Intensity and duration. If you have not been active and have not done any swimming for a long time, begin a swimming program by spending two or three weeks (three times per week) leisurely swimming at a pace that keeps your heart rate 10 to 20 percent below your EBZ. Gradually increase either the duration, the intensity, or both duration and intensity of your swimming to raise your heart rate to a comfortable level within your EBZ, as described below. This can be done by alternating swimming intervals with rest intervals and by gradually increasing the swimming intervals and decreasing the rest intervals.

Calories burned while swimming are the result of the pace: how far you swim and how fast (see Table 7–13).

Frequency. Swim at least three times per week (more often if you want changes in body composition).

At the beginning

Nonswimmers may need a good deal of instruction to develop the necessary skills. (But even the instructional program can be a valuable fitness experience for beginners, while at the same time teaching them swimming skills.)

A major factor in effective swimming is the ability to breathe rhythmically. With this technique, breathing is coordinated with the stroke—you inhale when your face is out of the water and exhale when your face is submerged. It takes a while for most beginners to learn rhythmic breathing. So if you're serious about your swimming—and if breathing while swimming is a problem for you—it will pay to invest the time and the money for instruction.

If you already know how to swim, and are ready to begin the model program, be sure to start each session with a ten-minute warm-up (see stretching model program).

Start swimming laps of the width of the pool if you can't swim the length. To keep your heart rate below your EBZ, take rest intervals as needed. Swim one lap and rest fifteen to ninety seconds as needed. Start with ten minutes of swim/rest intervals and work up to fifteen minutes. How long it will take you depends on your swimming skills and your muscular fitness.

As you progress

Once you can swim the length of the pool at a pace that now keeps your heart rate within your EBZ, continue swim/rest intervals for twenty minutes. The rest intervals should be thirty to forty-five seconds. You may find it helpful to get out of the pool during the rest interval and walk for the thirty to forty-five seconds, or until you've lowered your heart rate.

Next, swim two laps of the pool length and continue swim/rest intervals for thirty minutes. For the thirty-second rest interval between every two laps, walk (or rest) until you've lowered your heart rate. Gradually

154

increase the number of consecutive swimming laps until you feel ready to try to swim for fifteen minutes without stopping. Select a pace that allows you to keep your heart rate within your EBZ when swimming nonstop for fifteen minutes. At a pace of 20 yards per minute, you will swim about 300 yards; at a 45-yard-per-minute pace, you will cover about 1,000 yards in fifteen minutes. Be cautious about swimming at too fast a pace: It can take your heart rate too high and limit your ability to sustain your swimming.

Varying your strokes can rest your muscles and help prolong the swim. A variety of strokes will also involve more muscle groups and provide a better balanced workout.

Table 7–13

Determining Calorie Cost for Swimming

To use this Table, find on the horizontal line the distance in yards that most closely approximates the distance you swim. Next, locate on the appropriate vertical column (below the distance in yards) the time it takes you to swim the distance. Then locate in the first column on the left the approximate number of calories burned per minute per pound for the time and distance. To find the total number of calories burned, multiply your weight by the calories per minute per pound. Then multiply the product of these two numbers by the time it takes you to swim the distance (minutes:seconds). For example, assuming you weigh 154 pounds and swim 100 yards in 4 minutes, you would burn 25 calories: $154 \times .041$ (calories per pound, from Table) $= .63 \times 4$ (minutes) $= 25$ calories burned.

Calories per minute per pound	Distance in yards					
	25	100	150	250	500	750
.033	1:15	5:00	7:30	12:30	25:00	30:30
.041	1:00	4:00	6:00	10:00	20:00	30:00
.049	0:50	3:20	5:00	8:20	18:40	25:00
.057	0:43	2:52	4:18	7:10	17:20	21:30
.065	0:37.5	2:30	3:45	6:15	10:00	
.073	0:33	2:13	3:20	5:30	8:50	
.081	0:30	2:00	3:00	5:00	8:00	
.090	0:27	1:48	2:42	4:30	7:12	
.097	0:25	1:40	2:30	4:10	6:30	

Health and safety tips

■ Swim only in a pool with a qualified lifeguard on duty.

■ Dry your ears well after swimming. If you experience the symptoms of swimmer's ear (itching, discharge, or even a partial hearing loss), consult your physician. If you swim while recovering from swimmer's ear, protect your ears with a few drops of lanolin on a wad of lamb's wool.

Weight training

The most effective means for developing both muscular strength and muscular endurance is weight training—whether you use a weight training machine or simply barbells and dumbbells. And this model program of seven exercises will enhance the strength and endurance of all your major muscle groups. The model program requires you to select a weight for each of the seven exercises, performing at least 8 repetitions of each exercise. When you are able to perform 15 repetitions, you increase the weight.

This basic program in progressive weight training is suitable for almost everyone regardless of the level of muscular fitness. You can tailor the program to your level of strength by selecting the amount of resistance you can handle.

People with coronary heart disease, coronary risk factors, or circulatory ailments, however, should consult a physician before beginning a program in weight training. And it must be specially adapted for a person with orthopedic problems (see page 91).

Terminology

Here are the terms you'll need to know in doing this model program.

Load. The total number of pounds lifted during each movement of an exercise, including the weight of the bar, the plates, and the collars (see Equipment).

Resistance. A force tending to prevent motion: A 10-pound weight offers more resistance than a 5-pound weight. When you increase the resistance (by adding weight to the equipment), your muscles work harder. The harder they work, the stronger they become. This regular increase in resistance provides overload—and this is what results in progress.

Repetitions. The number of times you perform an exercise.

Set. A series of repetitions for a specific exercise.

Weight training program

Purpose. To develop and maintain muscular strength and endurance of the major muscle groups.

Equipment. Weight training requires its own unique equipment, usually available at sporting-goods stores. (Vinyl-covered weights won't scratch the floor but are bulkier than the cast iron variety and take up more room.)

■ Bar: A steel bar or pipe 4, 5, or 6 feet long. The middle section of the bar may have a knurled surface to provide friction for gripping.

■ Barbell: A bar with plates and collars attached.

■ Collars: Metal rings with set screws used to hold the plates in place on the bar.

■ Plates: Iron or sand-filled plastic discs with a center hole. These are slipped onto the ends of the bar and secured with collars. Plates are usually available in weights of 1¼, 2½, 5, 10, 20 pounds and up.

■ Bench: A bench 12 to 16 inches high, 10 to 16 inches wide, and 4 to 6 feet long, preferably padded; used for performing certain exercises.

Intensity and duration. Start with a load you can handle easily. Always attempt to do as many repetitions as you can—but not less than 8. Perform one set, rest, and perform another set of the same exercise; rest and perform a third set of the same exercise. Then move on to the next exercise. Continue until you have completed all seven exercises. When you can do three sets of 15 repetitions of an exercise, increase the load by adding weight. After each increase in load, return to performing three sets of as many repetitions as you can (but not less than 8). Keep on with this system during your workouts until you can perform three sets of 15 repetitions with the new load. Continue this progressive overloading, by increasing weight and repetitions, until you reach the level of strength and endurance you wish. To maintain the strength and endurance you have now achieved, exercise at that level of load and repetitions.

Frequency. Weight training fatigues the muscles, so it's wise to rest a day between workouts. If you wish, you may work out every day by exercising the upper body one day and the lower body the next. With this model program, we recommend that you work out every other day.

At the beginning

Always warm up by doing the "clean-and-press" with a weight light enough so you can easily perform from 10 to 15 repetitions. (Or use the warm-up/cool-down in the stretching model program.) By trial-and-error, establish for each exercise a load light enough to be lifted *with ease* for a set of 8 repetitions. Continue with this load for three to five workouts to allow the joints and muscles to make a gradual adjustment and to avoid soreness and stiffness.

It's a good idea to record the number of repetitions and the load you use at each workout. To do this, adapt Table 7–10, the sample progress chart in the interval circuit training model program.

As you progress

After you become proficient in weight training, you may want to progress beyond the model program—to work on some specific fitness goal, perhaps. If you want to concentrate on *muscular strength*, follow a program of 6 to 8 repetitions. Select a weight with which you can complete a minimum of 6 repetitions; when you can perform 8 repetitions, increase the weight and begin again at 6 repetitions. If you want to concentrate on *muscular endurance*, then follow a program of 15 to 25 repetitions. When you can perform 25 repetitions, increase the weight and begin again at 15 repetitions. To develop both muscular strength *and* muscular endurance, a system of from 8 to 15 repetitions would be appropriate.

Weight training can be helpful if you're interested in improving your sports performance. Study the sport to find out which of the muscle groups you should work on. You can then direct your weight training toward the development of the specific muscles involved.

Safety tips

■ Before you begin a workout, be sure the collars and plates are tightly secured.

■ Use a towel or chalk to keep your hands dry.

■ Avoid holding your breath while lifting weights. Get into the habit of inhaling in preparation for the lift and exhaling at the conclusion of the lift.

■ Do not lift heavy weights unless you're accompanied by two "spotters," who can help if you lose your balance.

Weight training exercises

Refer to the Glossary of Exercises for instructions on how to perform these exercises. For best results, do the exercises in the numerical sequence below. The body parts affected by the exercises are noted for each.

Warm-up: Clean and press
(See Glossary 4B)

Full body

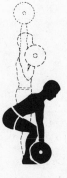

---

1. Curl
(See Glossary 7B)

Biceps, forearms

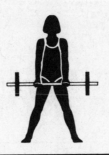

2. Military press
(See Glossary 5B)

Upper back, shoulders, arms

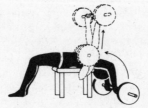

3. Bent rowing
(See Glossary 3B)

Upper back, arms

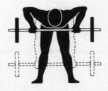

4. Bent-arm pull-over and press
(See Glossary 23B)

Upper back, chest, triceps

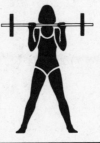

5. Parallel squat
(See Glossary 17B)

Quadriceps, hips

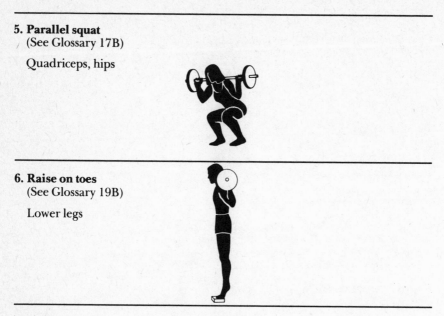

6. Raise on toes
(See Glossary 19B)

Lower legs

7. Sit-up
(See Glossary 24E)

Abdominals

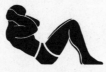

Home exercise equipment

For many exercisers, the fully equipped commercial gymnasium or the lure of the outdoors is exciting and stimulating. Fortunately, there's an alternative if you prefer privacy during your attempts to improve physical fitness: You can set aside space at home for exercising. In fact, most home exercisers don't need very much space. And some exercise programs don't even need any store-bought equipment at all. With ordinary items found in any home you can develop a circuit training program (based on the interval circuit training model program), which can benefit all the components of physical fitness (see Table 7–14).

Some households already have exercise equipment available. The stationary bicycle, for example, can form the basis for a useful circuit training program (see Table 7–15).

No equipment or program can provide fitness benefits, however, unless used correctly on a regular basis. The principles of progressive overload (intensity, duration, and frequency) and specificity must be observed. To develop and maintain physical fitness, a program using household items or equipment must meet certain criteria.

Cardiorespiratory endurance (CRE). Equipment is useful for CRE if it offers the opportunity to exercise within your EBZ for a minimum of fifteen minutes. Usually the exercise must involve the body's largest muscle groups—the legs (including thighs) and the back.

Body composition. Equipment for improving body composition must

---

Table 7–14

Circuit Training Using Household Items

The circuit below can last for durations ranging from 15 minutes to one hour by adjusting the number of trips around the circuit and the number of repetitions performed for each exercise. Follow the interval circuit training model program— 30 seconds of exercise followed by 15 seconds of rest. Refer to the Glossary of Exercises for explanations of how to perform most of the exercises. The final column notes the body parts affected by the exercises. CRE is improved by rope skipping and the step-up, as well as by the circuit as a whole.

Glossary number	Exercise	Equipment needed	Body parts affected
20F	Towel stretch	Towel	Triceps, shoulders, upper back
3E	Twister	Mop or broom handle	Hamstrings, trunk
25E	Push-up	2 chairs	Chest, triceps, upper back
24E	Sit-up	Sofa or dresser	Abdominals
—	Rope skipping	Clothesline	Lower legs
1D	Lateral raise	2 books	Shoulders
15F	Block stretch	Phone book	Lower legs
26E	Chin	Broomstick & 2 chairs	Upper back, chest, biceps
23E	Step-up	Stair or low stool	Thighs, hips

161

allow you to burn a high number of calories during one exercise session, which should last thirty minutes or more.

Muscular strength. To develop muscular strength, the equipment must be capable of supplying sufficient resistance for 6 to 8 repetitions during maximum effort.

Muscular endurance. Muscular endurance equipment must allow you to perform at least 15 repetitions, with the potential of increasing to 25 repetitions or more during maximum effort.

Flexibility. To be considered useful, equipment for improving flexibility must permit movement through the full range of motion of the joints.

Equipment for home exercise circuit

If you already have it on hand, you might like to use in a circuit training program the store-bought exercise equipment listed below (see Table 7–15).

Stationary exercise bicycle. In January 1982 *Consumer Reports* reported on a total of eighteen models of single-action stationary bicycles. Exercise on a single-action bike is pedaling, as on a regular bike. The stationary bike is capable of promoting CRE and muscular endurance of the leg muscles. By providing variable pedaling resistance to the needs of the exerciser, it can require sufficient effort of the large muscle groups of the legs to push the heart rate into the exercise benefit zone (EBZ). Because pedaling can burn a lot of calories, regular use should also contribute to the loss of body fat. Check your pulse rate regularly when you start the program to find out if you're pedaling hard enough to stay within your EBZ.

Another type of stationary exercise bike is the motorized model that generates a coordinated movement of the pedals, seat, and handlebars. It may operate at one or two rates of speed. The most productive way of using this model is to attempt to push, pull, and pedal as if to speed up the action—even though you really can't make it go faster.

If used regularly, the motorized stationary bike can develop CRE as well as many muscle groups. The most effective approach is use of an interval training system. For example, you may pull, push, and pedal for ten to fifteen seconds and then let the motor take over for fifteen to thirty seconds of relief interval. At first you may let the bike do much of the work. In time, however, you should find that the intensity and duration of active push, pull, and pedal intervals will increase.

Rowing machine. The rowing machine is designed to simulate the action of competitive rowing. Handles are available as "oars," usually with incre-

162

ments to decrease or increase resistance. The feet are generally strapped to foot rests to ensure strong leg action (particularly of the quadriceps but also of the hamstrings).

You can maintain your heart rate within your EBZ if you extend your legs vigorously and your arms and back are fully active. Vary the pace to ensure adequate intensity and duration. In addition to its CRE value, the rowing machine can develop muscular endurance in the arms, upper and lower back, and the legs. Rowing can also promote flexibility of most of the joints.

Allow time for your muscles to become conditioned to the movement of rowing. Begin with a few minutes of slow-paced rowing without con-

Table 7–15

Circuit Training Using Available Home Exercise Equipment

Although the circuit below focuses on a stationary bicycle, it could just as easily focus on a rowing machine, a nonmotorized treadmill, or a jump rope. This circuit can last for durations ranging from 15 minutes to one hour by adjusting the number of trips around the circuit and by increasing the time on the stationary bicycle. Follow the interval circuit training model program—30 seconds of exercise followed by 15 seconds of rest. If you want to emphasize CRE, increase each set of cycling: Instead of 30 seconds, do 2 to 5 minutes. (Use miles instead of repetitions for cycling.) Refer to the Glossary of Exercises for explanations of how to perform many of the exercises. The final column notes the body parts affected by the exercises. CRE is improved by cycling and by the circuit as a whole.

Glossary number	Exercise	Equipment needed	Body parts affected
—	Bicycling	Stationary bicycle	Legs, hips
3C	Overhead pull	Cables	Upper back, chest
24E	Sit-up	Slant board	Abdominals
—	Bicycling	Stationary bicycle	Legs, hips
2C	Archer's	Cables	Upper back, triceps
20E	Back extension	———	Lower back
—	Bicycling	Stationary bicycle	Legs, hips
25E	Push-up	———	Chest, triceps, upper back
—	Wrist flexion	Wrist roller	Wrists, forearms

163

cern for reaching your EBZ. At a comfortable rowing pace, gradually increase duration over a period of several weeks. Then try to reach your EBZ and to prolong your duration for a minimim of fifteen minutes.

If you have high blood pressure, or orthopedic or circulatory problems, you should get medical clearance before beginning an exercise program based on the rowing machine.

Treadmill. Motorized treadmills are expensive and are generally found only in university or college physical education laboratories, medical facilities, and commercial exercise facilities.

Nonmotorized treadmills cost far less and can provide partially adjustable inclines for jogging or walking uphill. The nonmotorized treadmill can be useful for developing CRE. Warming up with the basic stretching model, followed by weight training exercises or calisthenics, and finishing your program on the treadmill can give you a well-rounded exercise program. Like the stationary bicycle and rowing machine, the nonmotorized treadmill provides an opportunity for year-round CRE exercise regardless of the weather.

Jump rope. The jump rope, whether it is a fancy handled-model or just a piece of clothesline, is a useful device for developing CRE and muscular endurance of the lower legs. Because rope skipping is relatively high in calorie cost, it can improve body composition. (See rope skipping model program.)

Cables. Originally known as "chest expanders" and sometimes called "spring exercisers," this inexpensive piece of equipment may consist of as few as three and as many as ten strands of steel springs attached to handles. The device often comes with five springs that may be removed or added in order to adjust the resistance. Cables can develop muscular strength and muscular endurance of the arms, chest, shoulders, and upper back. Flexibility of the chest and shoulder muscles may be improved as well.

Slant board. Frequently called an abdominal board, the slant board increases resistance while doing sit-ups with the foot end of the board raised: The higher the angle, the greater the difficulty of the sit-up. The board can also be used for leg, hip, and back exercises. (By raising both ends of the board off the floor—by placing it on chairs, for instance—the slant board can serve as an exercise bench for weight training exercises.)

Wrist roller. This is an excellent device for developing muscular strength and muscular endurance of the wrists and forearms. Attach a rope to a 2-inch dowel (or broomstick). Tie a weight—a size you can handle easily —to the end of the rope. Hold the dowel with one hand at each end (with

164

the rope and weight in the center of the dowel). With your arms either horizontally straight in front of you or bent at the elbow, lower the weight by unwinding the rope, rotating the dowel away from the body. Then bring the weight back up by rewinding the rope around the dowel. Reverse the procedure to vary the exercise.

Other home exercise equipment

Not all home exercise equipment can become the focus for a circuit training program. But the kinds of home exercise equipment described below can be used to help you improve fitness.

Chest crusher. Very useful for developing the muscles of the chest (pectorals), the chest crusher also involves the biceps and shoulders to some extent. Sometimes erroneously called "a bust developer," it actually affects the muscles that serve as a foundation to and support for the breasts.

Chinning bar. This is a useful and inexpensive piece of equipment. Some store-bought types can be attached to the wall and others can be placed in a doorway (they telescope so require no screws or bolts). Another alternative is to mount a homemade bar in the rafters of your attic or in the basement.

Chinning exercises can enhance muscular strength and muscular endurance of the arms, chest, upper back, and trunk. Relaxed hanging by the hands (with some slow twisting and stretching) can improve flexibility of the shoulders and upper back. For a balanced program, CRE activities would also be necessary.

Doorknob exercise. This is a device that attaches to a doorknob with a pulley so that the exerciser can pull with one handle of the rope while resisting with the other. The value in terms of muscular strength and muscular endurance depends on the exerciser: Simply going through motions is a waste of time. But actively pulling and resisting can influence muscular endurance and to some extent muscular strength. The device has little or no value for any other fitness component.

Exercise wheel. The exercise wheel is a device that is marketed to "trim your tummy." If used properly, it can improve muscular strength and muscular endurance of your abdominal muscles, chest, and upper back. It will not result in spot reduction of body fat—there's no such thing (see page 80). But it will improve the firmness of your abdominal muscles.

The exercise wheel consists of a dowel used as an axle inserted through the center of a solid wheel (sometimes two wheels). Kneel on the floor so that the axle is in line with your shoulders and grasp the axle. Raising your head, inhale and extend your arms forward, rolling the wheel out as far as you can reach comfortably. Exhale slowly and hold the outstretched position for a second or two. Then inhale slowly as you roll the wheel back to starting position.

When first using this piece of equipment, limit the extent of the movement. (You could fall on your face.) It's also wise for a beginner to do only 3 to 5 repetitions to avoid muscle soreness. The exercise wheel forces the abdominal muscles to function as stabilizers of the trunk in a way that does not occur in most calisthenics.

Grip exerciser. This piece of equipment can develop the muscular strength and muscular endurance of your grip—depending on the tension of the particular model. If your sports interest requires strong wrists and forearms, as in tennis or handball, this device may be helpful.

Some people keep a grip exerciser in their car and use it when caught in traffic or at stop lights. (It can be an effective way to release tension.) Others use it while watching television or riding a stationary bicycle.

8

Sports and Activities

If you're a novice at exercise, model programs are a perfect way to get you started on improving your level of fitness. They benefit one or more of the five fitness components and can help you make progress toward achieving your fitness goals. For more experienced exercisers, however, and for those who have done the model programs and now want to supplement the routine with other less-structured forms of exercise, this chapter presents an overview of some eighty sports and activities to choose from.

Table 8–1 is a summary list of the sports and activities covered in Chapters 7 and 8. They are classified on the basis of their potential for developing each of the five fitness components. These classifications are guidelines: Certain activities may be more (or less) valuable because of differing skills, personal styles of play, and the stamina one has to keep at a sport or activity longer than usual. Also noted in the Table are the skill levels required to obtain fitness benefits from the activity, the fitness prerequisite needed for participation, and how the activity is paced. Following the Table are brief discussions of sports and activities, including for most of them a chart summarizing the activity's potential for achieving each of the five fitness components and, where appropriate, the parts of the body affected (the parts most affected are listed first). Also shown in the charts for activities that provide CRE and body composition benefits is an estimate of the number of calories you burn per pound per minute.

If the sport or activity you choose is designed to improve CRE and body composition, it would be helpful to keep track of the calories you burn. To do so, use the "Estimating calorie cost" section of the chart to get an approximate total. On many of the charts you get a choice of calorie figures—for moderate or for vigorous exercise, say. Use whichever is more appropriate to calculate the calories burned. For example, if the chart shows that a sport or activity burns .039 calories (for moderate

167

exercise) per minute per pound and you weigh 140 pounds and you exercise for thirty minutes, the formula is: .039 × 140 × 30 = 164 calories burned.

Do not be misled by the seeming precision of the calorie estimates. In many cases, they represent a "best guess," based on available research supplemented by the experience of our senior authors and other authorities.

Explanation of fitness components ratings

The classifications of low (L), moderate (M), and high (H) for the five components of physical fitness are based on the ability of a sport or activity to develop that component.

Cardiorespiratory endurance (CRE). Each sport or activity is classified for its potential value in promoting CRE. Those classified as high in CRE are the kind that can maintain the heart rate in the exercise benefit zone (EBZ, see pages 62–66) for at least fifteen minutes. If the activity is self-paced as well, it would be an excellent foundation for a CRE program.

An activity classified as high in CRE but paced by others—either because of competition or an exercise leader—can also maintain the heart rate in the EBZ for periods of time. But because the pacing is not individualized, the heart rate may be driven above (or drop below) the EBZ for some participants. Such a sport or activity, while useful for developing CRE, should not replace a self-paced, high-CRE sport or activity as the mainstay of a fitness program.

At the other extreme, a sport or activity classified as low in CRE is one that is either anaerobic (see page 54), or of such low intensity that it cannot generally raise the heart rate into the EBZ. For a low-intensity sport or activity to raise the heart rate into the EBZ and thus accrue CRE benefits would require more than an hour's continuous active participation.

A sport or activity is classified as moderate, whether it's self-paced or competitively paced, because although heart rate can be brought into the EBZ, it's difficult to maintain it there for at least fifteen minutes. However, a moderate CRE activity—with its alternating periods in and out of the EBZ—can be a form of interval training, as long as the periods when the heart rate is in the EBZ last for at least two minutes at a time.

Body composition (BC). Body composition, particularly reduction in body fat, is best influenced by sports or activities that are classified high in CRE. However, sports or activities classified high, or even moderate, for developing muscular endurance also help to improve body composition.

Muscular strength (MS), muscular endurance (ME), and flexibility (F). For someone interested in developing muscular strength and muscular endurance, weight training is the ideal activity. It's classified high for both fitness components. A weight trainer can control the activity to a high degree and realize the potential for progressive overload by using the exact amount of weight needed to perform the repetitions required to achieve either or both muscular strength or muscular endurance. (See weight training model program in Chapter 7.)

If weight training is not feasible, there are other activities classified as high for development of muscular strength or muscular endurance. See, for example, the interval circuit training model program and calisthenic circuit training model program in Chapter 7, and isotonics, isometrics, and isokinetics in Chapter 5.

Yoga is an example of an activity high in flexibility. It puts all muscle groups and joints through a full range of movement and enables you to provide progressive overload easily and comfortably. Other activities high in flexibility include modern dance and gymnastics.

Table 8–1

Summary of Sports and Activities

This Table lists the sports and activities included in Chapters 7 and 8, classifying them as high (H), moderate (M), or low (L) in terms of their ability to develop each of the five components of physical fitness. (See page 168 for an explanation of the system of classification.) The skill level needed to obtain fitness benefits is noted: low (L) means little or no skill is required to obtain fitness benefits; moderate (M) means average skill is needed to obtain fitness benefits; and high (H) means much skill is required to obtain fitness benefits. The fitness prerequisite—conditioning needs of a beginner—is also noted: low (L) means no fitness prerequisite is required; moderate (M) means some preconditioning is required; and high (H) means substantial fitness is required. In the last column, each sport and activity is rated in terms of how it's paced: 1 means it's self-paced; 2 means it's a combination of self and others; and 3 means it's paced by someone other than yourself.

Sports and activities	Components					Skill level	Fitness prerequisite	How paced
	CRE	BC	MS	ME	F			
Aerobic dance	H	H	M	H	H	L	L	3
Aqua exercises	L	L	M	M	M	L	L	1
Archery	L	L	L	L	L	L	L	1
Backpacking	H	H	H	H	M	L	M	1
Badminton (skilled, singles)	H	H	M	M	M	M	M	2
Balance beam	L	M	H	H	H	H	H	1

Sports and activities	Components					Skill level	Fitness prerequisite	How paced
	CRE	BC	MS	ME	F			
Ballet (floor combinations)	M	M	M	H	H	M	L	3
Ballroom dancing	M	M	L	M	L	M	L	3
Baseball (pitcher & catcher)	M	M	M	H	M	H	M	3
Basketball	H	H	M	H	M	M	M	3
Bicycling	H	H	M	H	M	M	L	1
Bowling	L	L	L	L	L	L	L	1
Boxing	H	H	M	H	M	M	M	2
Calisthenic circuit training	H	H	M	H	M	L	L	1
Canoeing & kayaking	M	M	M	H	M	M	M	1
Cheerleading	M	M	M	M	M	M	L	3
Cross-country skiing	H	H	M	H	M	M	M	1
Disco dancing	M	M	L	M	M	M	L	3
Diving/springboard	L	L	M	M	H	H	M	1
Fencing	M	M	M	H	H	M	L	3
Field hockey	H	H	M	H	M	M	M	3
Fishing	L	L	L	L	L	L	L	1
Folk & square dancing	M	M	L	M	L	L	L	3
Football/touch	M	M	M	M	M	M	M	3
Frisbee/ultimate	H	H	M	H	M	M	M	2
Golf (riding cart)	L	L	L	L	M	L	L	1
Handball (skilled, singles)	H	H	M	H	M	M	M	3
High bar	L	M	H	H	H	H	H	1
Hiking	H	H	M	H	L	L	M	1
Hockey/ice & roller	H	H	M	H	M	M	M	3
Horseback riding	M	M	M	M	L	M	M	1
Hunting	L	L	L	M	L	L	M	1
Interval circuit training	H	H	H	H	M	L	L	1
Jogging & running	H	H	M	H	L	L	L	1
Judo	M	M	H	H	M	M	L	3
Jumping/track & field	L	M	H	M	H	M	L	1
Karate	H	H	M	H	H	L	M	3
Lacrosse	H	H	M	H	M	H	M	3
Modern dance (moving combinations)	M	M	M	H	H	L	L	3
Orienteering	H	H	M	H	L	L	M	1

Sports and activities	Components CRE	BC	MS	ME	F	Skill level	Fitness prerequisite	How paced
Outdoor fitness trails	H	H	M	H	M	L	L	1
Paddleball (skilled, singles)	H	H	M	H	M	M	M	2
Paddle tennis (skilled, singles)	H	H	M	M	M	M	M	2
Parallel bars	L	M	H	H	H	H	H	1
Platform tennis (skilled, singles)	H	H	M	M	M	M	M	2
Pole vault	L	M	H	M	H	H	H	1
Racquetball (skilled, singles)	H	H	M	M	M	M	M	2
Rock climbing	M	M	H	H	H	H	M	1
Rope skipping	H	H	M	H	L	M	M	1
Rowing	H	H	H	H	H	L	L	1
RCAF program (5BX & XBX)	M	M	M	H	M	L	L	1
Rugby	H	H	M	H	M	M	M	3
Sailing	L	L	L	M	L	M	L	1
Scuba diving	M	M	M	H	M	H	M	1
Side horse	L	M	M	H	H	H	H	1
Skateboarding	M	M	M	M	M	H	M	1
Skating/ice & roller	M	M	M	H	M	H	M	1
Skiing/Alpine	M	M	H	H	M	H	M	1
Skin diving	M	M	M	H	M	M	M	1
Snowshoeing	H	H	M	H	M	L	L	1
Soccer	H	H	M	H	M	M	M	3
Sprinting	L	M	H	M	M	L	M	1
Squash (skilled, singles)	H	H	M	M	M	M	M	2
Stretching/warm-up & cool-down	L	L	L	L	H	L	L	1
Surfboarding	M	M	M	M	M	H	M	2
Swimming	H	H	M	H	M	M	L	1
Synchronized swimming	M	M	M	H	H	H	M	3
Table tennis	M	M	L	M	M	M	L	3
Tai Chi Chuan	L	L	L	M	M	M	L	1
Team handball	H	H	M	H	M	M	M	3
Tennis (skilled, singles)	H	H	M	M	M	M	M	2
Throwing/track & field	L	M	H	H	M	M	M	1
Trampoline	L	M	M	H	M	M	M	1
Tumbling	L	M	H	H	H	H	M	1

Sports and activities	Components					Skill level	Fitness prerequisite	How paced
	CRE	BC	MS	ME	F			
Twirling/baton	M	M	M	H	H	H	M	1
Volleyball	M	M	L	M	M	M	M	3
Walking	H	H	L	M	L	L	L	1
Water polo	H	H	M	H	M	H	M	3
Waterskiing	M	M	M	H	M	H	M	2
Weight training	L	M	H	H	H	L	L	1
Wrestling	H	H	H	H	H	H	H	3
Yoga	L	L	L	M	H	H	L	1

Listing of sports and activities

The remainder of this chapter contains additional information about the sports and activities listed in Table 8–1. For some, only the chart portion appears, giving the classifications for each of the five components of physical fitness, and also the body parts affected and calorie information (where relevant). For most sports and activities, the chart is followed by a brief discussion of the exercise.

Aerobic dance (see also Dance)

Action	CRE	BC	MS	ME	F	Body parts affected
Moderate to vigorous	H	H	M	H	H	Legs, trunk

Estimating calorie cost

Moderate: **.046** × your weight × total minutes in action = approximate calories burned

Vigorous: **.062** × your weight × total minutes in action = approximate calories burned

Aerobic dance is a form of exercise that consists of thirty to sixty consecutive minutes of rhythmic running, hopping, skipping, jumping, sliding, stretching, and bending. It's performed to music and in response to directions called by an instructor in the manner of a square dance caller.

Classes are usually structured so that slow warm-up and stretching routines begin the session, followed by energetic and strenuous routines, and ending with slow cool-down routines. In a typical aerobic dance class,

172

participants work at varying intensities with periodic breaks for checking the pulse. A person with low CRE can walk through some routines or do fewer repetitions while gradually building up the skill required to execute the steps and the CRE to do them at jogging or running intensities.

Aerobic dance can provide a high level of conditioning of most fitness components. It can affect the entire body, including the cardiorespiratory system. It can be the foundation of your fitness program, or provide supplemental or substitute workouts in a regimen consisting of several activities. Once you learn the routines, you can practice them at home to the music of a radio, tapes, or a record player.

A variation on aerobic dance is Jazzercise—exercises and dance steps combined into a series of dance sequences. It too can be performed at home once you learn the basic exercises and dance steps.

Aqua exercises

CRE	BC	MS	ME	F	Body parts affected
L	L	M	M	M	Full body

Aqua exercises, often refered to as water calisthenics, can be a pleasant and entertaining activity. When submerged in water, the body experiences an exhilaration associated with moderate increases in blood circulation and deep breathing. But more significant, water is a buoyant force: A one-hundred-fifty-pound person exercising in water, for example, feels as if only fifteen pounds were being exercised. Not having to work against gravity is a particularly useful way to exercise for those who have been sedentary or who suffer from muscle or joint injuries.

Aqua exercises, depending on how they're done, develop three fitness components. Moving against the resistance of water is isokinetic exercise (see Chapter 5) and can help build muscular strength and endurance. It's also much easier to stretch in water, thereby promoting flexibility.

While aqua exercises may provide a simple, comfortable way to exercise, it's still wise to ease into a program, increasing intensity and duration at increments that allow your muscles to become gradually adjusted to the activity. Refer to the aqua exercises illustrated in the Glossary of Exercises for suggestions on how to utilize a pool to develop your own program. After a few weeks, you will be able to select calisthenic exercises from the Glossary to adapt for use in the water and to design new exercises—ones that feel good to you.

Archery

CRE	BC	MS	ME	F	Body parts affected
L	L	L	L	L	Arms, shoulders

173

Archery dates back to olden times when it was used to obtain food and as a weapon of war. Over the years, it has evolved into a recreational sport ranging from a backyard activity that can be fun for the entire family to hunting with a crossbow and Olympic competition. Archery is primarily a matter of motor skill, particularly eye/hand coordination. Thus it does little to improve most fitness components. It affects only the arms and shoulders.

Backpacking (*see also* Hiking)

Action	CRE	BC	MS	ME	F	Body parts affected
With 40-lb. pack	H	H	H	H	M	Hips, thighs, lower legs, shoulders, abdominals

Estimating calorie cost

3 mph, level terrain: **.032** × your weight × total minutes in action = approximate calories burned

3.5 mph, 5° grade: **.052** × your weight × total minutes in action = approximate calories burned

3.5 mph, 15° grade: **.078** × your weight × total minutes in action = approximate calories burned

1.5 mph, 36° grade: **.103** × your weight × total minutes in action = approximate calories burned

Backpackers go hiking for more than one day at a time, carrying supplies and equipment for overnight camping in packs that may weigh twenty-five pounds or more. Like any sort of hiking, backpacking is a way to improve CRE, body composition, and muscular strength and endurance. Flexibility of the hips, knees, and ankles is an extra benefit when you hike in mountainous areas.

Beginners can benefit from a course in backpacking, either from a backpackers' club or at a local college or other institution. And plan on going out with experienced backpackers for several hikes. Try to go on a trip with no less than four people. If someone is injured, one person can remain with the injured person, while the other two seek help.

Look through some catalogs and visit stores that carry outdoor equipment before you begin to buy the equipment you need. Don't wear new boots until they're broken in to the point that they are comfortable to wear for long stretches of time. When backpacking, be sure to drink plenty of water to avoid dehydration. And, of course, give family or friends your planned trip route and schedule.

The weight of the backpack makes some preconditioning a good idea. To prepare yourself for your first hike, begin a walking or jogging model program—and give up elevators for several weeks. Neck, shoulder, and abdominal exercises will also help.

Badminton (*see also* Racquet, wall & net sports)

Action	CRE	BC	MS	ME	F	Body parts affected
Skilled, singles	H	H	M	M	M	Legs
Beginner, singles; all doubles	M	M	L	L	M	Legs

Estimating calorie cost

Beginner: .032 × your weight × total minutes in action = approximate calories burned

Skilled, doubles: .042 × your weight × total minutes in action = approximate calories burned

Skilled, singles: .071 × your weight × total minutes in action = approximate calories burned

Badminton can be played indoors or out, as either singles or doubles. Indoor badminton courts can be found in schools and colleges. The outdoor game is usually played on an improvised backyard court where the family gets together to hit back and forth over the net a lightweight shuttlecock (made of cork with feathers on it). It's a game that people of all ages can play so long as they are fairly active. When played by highly skilled competitors, it is an exceedingly strenuous activity.

Balance beam (*see also* Gymnastics)

	CRE	BC	MS	ME	F	Body parts affected
	L	M	H	H	H	Legs, hips, trunk

Ballet (*see also* Dance)

Action	CRE	BC	MS	ME	F	Body parts affected
Barre	L	M	M	H	H	Legs, hips, trunk, arms
Floor combinations	M	M	M	H	H	Legs, hips, trunk, arms

Estimating calorie cost

Floor combinations: .058 × your weight × total minutes in action = approximate calories burned

Ballroom dancing (*see also* Dance)

175

Action	CRE	BC	MS	ME	F	Body parts affected
Moderate to vigorous	M	M	L	M	L	Legs, hips

Estimating calorie cost

Moderate: $.034 \times$ your weight $\times$ total minutes in action = approximate calories burned

Vigorous: $.049 \times$ your weight $\times$ total minutes in action = approximate calories burned

Baseball & softball

Action	CRE	BC	MS	ME	F	Body parts affected
Pitcher & catcher	M	M	M	H	M	Arms, shoulders, legs
Other players	L	L	M	M	L	Arms, shoulders, legs

Estimating calorie cost

Pitcher & catcher: $.039 \times$ your weight $\times$ total minutes in action = approximate calories burned

Unless you get to pitch three times per week or are the regular catcher on a team that plays almost daily, baseball can do little or nothing to improve most fitness components. Softball is just as unlikely to produce significant training effects. There is simply too much waiting around, either to field a ball or for your turn at bat. The brief spurts of intense activity are too limited to improve any of the fitness components.

People who are seriously involved in the game may, of course, participate in training programs that include jogging, weight training, calisthenics, and skill drills. It is these routines that upgrade the players' fitness as well as improve their playing effectiveness.

Basketball (*see also* Team sports)

Action	CRE	BC	MS	ME	F	Body parts affected
Moderate to vigorous, half court or full court	H	H	M	H	M	Arms, hips, quadriceps, hamstrings, lower legs

Estimating calorie cost

Moderate, half court: $.045 \times$ your weight $\times$ total minutes in action = approximate calories burned

Moderate, full court: $.052 \times$ your weight $\times$ total minutes in action = approximate calories burned

Vigorous, half court: $.071 \times$ your weight $\times$ total minutes in action = approximate calories burned

Vigorous, full court: .097 × your weight × total minutes in action =
                          approximate calories burned

Bicycling (*see also* bicycling model program in Chapter 7)

Action	CRE	BC	MS	ME	F	Body parts affected
10 to 13 mph	H	H	M	H	M	Legs, hips

Estimating calorie cost

10 mph: .049 × your weight × total minutes in action =
                          approximate calories burned

13 mph: .071 × your weight × total minutes in action =
                          approximate calories burned

Bowling

	CRE	BC	MS	ME	F	Body parts affected
	L	L	L	L	L	Bowling arm, wrist, shoulders

Bowling is as much a social event as a sport. It may be fun and good recreation, but it is of minimal value as a fitness exercise. It involves only intermittent, mild activity, usually interspersed with periods of sitting around and often punctuated with bouts of eating and drinking. A bowler's heart rate does not climb much beyond resting levels, so bowling is of little value as a CRE activity or to change body composition. Muscular strength in the bowling arm may be enhanced to a slight extent; so may flexibility in the lower back, if the bowler uses a crouched starting position. Otherwise, the benefits of bowling are almost entirely social and recreational.

Boxing

Action	CRE	BC	MS	ME	F	Body parts affected
Moderate to vigorous	H	H	M	H	M	Full body

Estimating calorie cost

Moderate: .052 × your weight × total minutes in action =
                          approximate calories burned

Vigorous: .078 × your weight × total minutes in action =
                          approximate calories burned

A boxer needs a high degree of all-around fitness to withstand the grueling punishment that the sport can inflict. The arduous training

177

regimen of the serious boxer usually involves plenty of rope skipping, running, sparring, and practice with punching bags. These activities develop high levels of muscular endurance in the arms and legs as well as the excellent CRE required to remain in competition. The light punching bag, commonly called the speed bag, has particularly good potential for developing high levels of CRE and muscular endurance of the arms. It must be used, however, as serious boxers use it, for ten to thirty minutes daily. But you don't have to be a boxer to incorporate the speed bag into a general fitness program. And all you need is an active imagination to include shadow boxing (against an invisible opponent) as another form of CRE exercise. If practiced for fifteen minutes or longer at high intensity, these two exercise routines can make valuable contributions to CRE as well as to muscular endurance.

Calisthenic circuit training (*see also* calisthenic circuit training model program in Chapter 7)

Action	CRE	BC	MS	ME	F	Body parts affected
3 sets or 20 min.	H	H	M	H	M	Full body

Estimating calorie cost

3 sets or 20 min.:   .06 × your weight × total minutes in action = approximate calories burned

Canoeing & kayaking

Action	CRE	BC	MS	ME	F	Body parts affected
Flat water, 2.5 to 4 mph	M	M	M	H	M	Arms, chest, shoulders

Estimating calorie cost

Flat water, 4 mph:*   .045 × your weight × total minutes in action = approximate calories burned

Canoeing differs from kayaking in the construction of the craft, the type of paddles, and how the paddles are used. The typical North American canoe is an open, rounded, hollow craft in which you kneel and paddle with a single blade. The kayak is usually smaller, lighter, and narrower and you sit while paddling alternately with the two blades of the paddle.

The fitness level you need to use a canoe or kayak, and the fitness benefits you get, can vary widely. Leisurely lake paddling requires some upper-body strength and endurance. If, however, you paddle a canoe or

---

*Much higher for competitive white-water canoeing.

kayak at a pace of 4 miles per hour for thirty minutes or more, you will probably find that your heart rate is in the EBZ and that significant CRE benefits can accrue. Extended outings on the water, particularly when they involve negotiating turbulent waters, or extensive training for competition requires not only high levels of fitness but considerable skill as well.

Cheerleading

Action	CRE	BC	MS	ME	F	Body parts affected
Moderate to vigorous	M	M	M	M	M	Full body

Estimating calorie cost

Moderate: **.033** × your weight × total minutes in action = approximate calories burned

Vigorous: **.049** × your weight × total minutes in action = approximate calories burned

Cheerleading usually conjures up an image of high school or college students vigorously leading spectators through rhythmic chants and yells at competitive athletic events. While the focus is on the prowess of the teams being cheered on to victory, the cheerleaders too need to be fit to perform their type of dance and gymnastics activities effectively. Cheerleading at games is sporadic so it may provide only limited fitness benefits. But the regular practice sessions are usually vigorous enough for development of all five fitness components.

Cross-country skiing

Action	CRE	BC	MS	ME	F	Body parts affected
3 to 8 mph	H	H	M	H	M	Full body

Estimating calorie cost

3 mph: **.049** × your weight × total minutes in action = approximate calories burned

8 mph: **.104** × your weight × total minutes in action = approximate calories burned

Competitive cross-country skiing is one of the most arduous athletic activities known. Some of the highest oxygen consumption levels have been recorded among cross-country skiers. Practiced on a regular basis, this activity has great potential for enhancing CRE and muscular endurance as well as body composition and muscular strength. Flexibility may

179

be increased in some joints. But in general, stretching exercises are advisable both as a warm-up activity and to balance the skiing program. Cross-country skiing is most enjoyable if you are already in good shape and know how to ski. However, since it is self-paced, it can produce a training effect as long as you ski on a regular basis and gradually increase the duration, intensity, and frequency of your outings.

This form of skiing can be performed wherever there is snow. Golf courses, woods, fields, snowmobile trails, and parks are all excellent terrains that require no ski lifts or fees. For your first outing, it's best to go with an experienced skier. If you begin at a pace that is comfortable for you, after an hour or two you will find that you can move along easily. By the end of the day, you should have developed at least a modicum of skills in cross-country skiing. You increase intensity with pace and by climbing hills. Brief downhill runs serve as pleasant relief intervals.

Dance (see also Aerobic dance, Ballet, Ballroom dancing, Disco dancing, Folk & square dancing, Modern dance)

The fitness benefits of dance vary considerably, depending on the particular dance forms. Dancers who practice jumps or leaps develop muscular strength, while those who practice extensive stretching, as in ballet and modern dance, have an excellent chance to develop flexibility. Muscular development of the upper body is limited, except in ballet and modern dance, which use the arms extensively in movement and for support for oneself or others.

CRE benefits vary in much the same way. A ballet or modern dance class usually begins with warm-up exercises, continues with a period of stretching and skill development, and concludes with the combination of various steps and movements to form a dance sequence or pattern. Only if these combinations are vigorous and long-lasting enough to put the heart rate into the EBZ and keep it there will there be CRE benefits. By contrast, folk dance enthusiasts who can perform a polka or a reel for fifteen or twenty minutes at a time are apt to maintain high levels of CRE.

The recent development of dance exercise specifically intended to improve physical fitness has added such forms as aerobic dance, Jazzercise, Slimnastics, and Dancercise to the repertoire. These methods are becoming increasingly available at "Y" associations, universities, and other institutions, as well as dance studios.

Disco dancing (see also Dance)

Action	CRE	BC	MS	ME	F	Body parts affected
Vigorous	M	M	L	M	M	Legs, hips

Estimating calorie cost

Vigorous: **.049** × your weight × total minutes in action = approximate calories burned

Diving/springboard

	CRE	BC	MS	ME	F	Body parts affected
	L	L	M	M	H	Trunk, legs

Skilled springboard diving requires and develops good levels of full-body flexibility as well as moderate to good levels of strength and endurance in the legs. These benefits are the result of frequent, lengthy practice sessions in which divers repeatedly take off from the diving board, swim to the pool side, vault out of the water, and climb to the board again. Such practice sessions may have CRE value if the diving/swimming sequence is conducted continuously, with little rest in between dives. Divers who are interested in developing CRE, however, should add extended periods of swimming to their diving practice sessions.

Fencing

Action	CRE	BC	MS	ME	F	Body parts affected
Moderate to vigorous	M	M	M	H	H	Fencing wrist, arm, shoulders, legs, hips

Estimating calorie cost

Moderate, drill: **.032** × your weight × total minutes in action = approximate calories burned

Vigorous, match: **.078** × your weight × total minutes in action = approximate calories burned

Fencing, whether with foil, épée, or saber, requires and develops muscular endurance and flexibility of the wrists, arms, and legs. It may also call for CRE if competition includes periods of intense offensive and defensive activity. These highly active bouts usually alternate with less active periods of sparring and brief intervals of rest. If continued for extended sessions, such interval training can, of course, result in CRE benefits.

Field hockey (*see also* Team sports)

Action	CRE	BC	MS	ME	F	Body parts affected
Moderate to vigorous	H	H	M	H	M	Legs, arms, trunk

181

Estimating calorie cost

Moderate: .052 × your weight × total minutes in action = approximate calories burned

Vigorous: .078 × your weight × total minutes in action = approximate calories burned

Fishing

CRE	BC	MS	ME	F
L	L	L	L	L

    Unless you have a long way to walk before beginning to fish, or unless you have to stalk the fish along a stream or a coastline, there is little about fishing to promote fitness. For deep-sea fishing, it can be especially helpful to have strength and endurance in the arms and hands if you have to contend with a powerful opponent at the other end of the line in a hard and long-lasting fight.

Folk & square dancing (*see also* Dance)

Action	CRE	BC	MS	ME	F	Body parts affected
Moderate to vigorous	M	M	L	M	L	Legs, hips

Estimating calorie cost

Moderate: .039 × your weight × total minutes in action = approximate calories burned

Vigorous: .049 × your weight × total minutes in action = approximate calories burned

Football/touch (*see also* Team sports)

Action	CRE	BC	MS	ME	F	Body parts affected
Moderate to vigorous	M	M	M	M	M	Legs, trunk

Estimating calorie cost

Moderate: .049 × your weight × total minutes in action = approximate calories burned

Vigorous: .078 × your weight × total minutes in action = approximate calories burned

Frisbee/ultimate (*see also* Team sports)

Action	CRE	BC	MS	ME	F	Body parts affected
Moderate to vigorous, team	H	H	M	H	M	Legs, arms

Estimating calorie cost

Moderate, team:	**.049** × your weight × total minutes in action = approximate calories burned
Vigorous, team:	**.078** × your weight × total minutes in action = approximate calories burned

Frisbee is the trade name for a saucer-shaped plastic disc that, when tossed, sails through the air. Tossing a Frisbee to and fro can lend itself to a variety of games and activities, with a wide range of potential fitness benefits. Leisurely tossing of a Frisbee yields relatively low fitness benefits. Games such as "Ultimate Frisbee," however, use the disc actively, in the manner of basketball, field hockey, soccer, or team handball, and can yield high CRE benefits. The bending and stretching required in running and jumping for a Frisbee help to promote flexibility as well. But unless you are interested and skillful enough to participate in one of the more vigorous organized Frisbee games, it's unlikely that tossing a Frisbee can serve as the basis for a fitness program.

Golf

Action	CRE	BC	MS	ME	F	Body parts affected
Riding cart	L	L	L	L	M	Legs, arms, shoulders, neck, trunk
Twosome pulling clubs, or foursome carrying clubs	L	L	M	M	M	Legs, arms, shoulders, neck, trunk
Twosome carrying clubs	M	M	M	M	M	Legs, arms, shoulders, neck, trunk

Estimating calorie cost

Twosome carrying clubs:	**.045** × your weight × total minutes in action = approximate calories burned

Golf requires skill and precision but is of limited fitness value. One authoritative study has shown that average golfers spend more than half their time on the course standing around—burning very few calories. About one-third of the time is spent walking (if not riding a cart); slightly less than 10 percent is spent actually swinging a club. How intense a CRE workout your golf game gives you depends on whether you ride a cart or walk; use a caddy, pull a golf bag, or carry your own clubs; whether you play in a foursome, in a twosome, or as a single; whether the course is flat or hilly; and how fast you play the game. Most golfers, even those who play over twelve hours per week, show no appreciable superiority in CRE over sedentary people who get no exercise at all. If, however, you play several times a week, alone or in a twosome, walk the course briskly, carry your own clubs, and avoid delays on the course, you may get CRE and weight control benefits from golf—the same as you would get from any vigorous three- or four-mile walk.

Swinging a golf club 68 to 100 or more times a round, twice or more a week, does little to increase muscular strength or endurance, although it may have some effect on flexibility of the shoulders, neck, and trunk. Serious golfers often take up weight training to increase their strength and to enhance the explosive power of their swing. Nonetheless, golf remains a relatively ineffective means of improving most of the components of physical fitness.

Gymnastics (see also Balance beam, High bar, Parallel bars, Side horse, Trampoline, Tumbling)

Gymnastics is a fast-growing sport, with programs available in many schools, "Y" associations, and specialized clubs. Because gymnastics requires the use of the entire body in twisting, turning, leaping, pushing, and pulling movements, it is an excellent way to improve and maintain muscular fitness. Gymnastics includes a variety of events using apparatus such as the side horse, long horse, trampoline, balance beam, parallel bars, and high bar, as well as other events, such as tumbling and free floor exercise, that use only mats. It is by performing a sequence of events that you can benefit from a gymnastics program.

Women's gymnastics puts greater emphasis on flexibility and dance-type movements while men's gymnastics puts greater emphasis on strength. Training is arduous, with the gymnast constantly working against his or her body weight. There is outstanding development of muscular strength, muscular endurance, and flexibility. And when the gymnast works continuously at a relatively high intensity for one or two hours, there are also CRE benefits.

Handball (see also Racquet, wall & net sports)

Action	CRE	BC	MS	ME	F	Body parts affected
Skilled, singles	H	H	M	H	M	Arms, shoulders, legs
Beginner, singles; all doubles	M	M	M	M	M	Arms, shoulders, legs

Estimating calorie cost

Beginner, singles; all doubles:	.049 × your weight × total minutes in action = approximate calories burned

184

Skilled, singles: **.078** × your weight × total minutes in action =
                              approximate calories burned

Inexpensive, widely available, and easy to master, handball is a popular sport. It can be played indoors or out, as singles or doubles, and with one, three, or four walls. When played at high intensity by skilled players, handball is a good way to achieve and maintain CRE and muscular endurance. Played long enough and frequently enough, it can affect body composition and be useful in weight control.

High bar (*see also* Gymnastics)

CRE	BC	MS	ME	F	Body parts affected
L	M	H	H	H	Shoulders, arms, trunk

Hiking (*see also* Backpacking, Orienteering)

Action	CRE	BC	MS	ME	F	Body parts affected
2 mph with a 10-lb. pack, 10° to 20° grade	H	H	M	H	L	Hips, thighs, lower legs, shoulders, abdominals

Estimating calorie cost

2 mph, 10° grade: **.051** × your weight × total minutes in action =
                              approximate calories burned

2 mph, 20° grade: **.073** × your weight × total minutes in action =
                              approximate calories burned

Hiking is walking with a view. It generally means taking a daylong excursion, out and back, with a little food, drink, and emergency gear carried in a light pack. The activity is self-paced, and only minimum fitness is required to begin. The fitness benefits of hiking are similar to those of walking. Distance, difficulty of terrain, and pace may be increased as fitness improves. It is wise to obtain information about trails and equipment needs beforehand and to leave your itinerary, including time schedule, with your family or friends.

Hockey/ice & roller (*see also* Team sports)

Action	CRE	BC	MS	ME	F	Body parts affected
Moderate to vigorous	H	H	M	H	M	Legs, arms

Estimating calorie cost

Moderate: **.052** × your weight × total minutes in action =
                              approximate calories burned

185

Vigorous: $.078 \times$ your weight $\times$ total minutes in action = approximate calories burned

Horseback riding

Action	CRE	BC	MS	ME	F	Body parts affected
Trot to gallop	M	M	M	M	L	Legs, trunk

Estimating calorie cost

Trot: $.052 \times$ your weight $\times$ total minutes in action = approximate calories burned

Gallop: $.065 \times$ your weight $\times$ total minutes in action = approximate calories burned

Being fit may be an asset to a rider, but leisurely horseback riding provides few fitness benefits to anyone except the horse. Riding a horse at a walk is a low-calorie activity. As the pace increases, however, so too does the involvement of the rider's legs and trunk, thereby increasing the energy cost. Thus trotting and galloping may offer CRE benefits to the burden as well as to the beast. Vigorous riding for long durations can also help to develop muscular endurance of the legs and trunk.

Hunting

	CRE	BC	MS	ME	F	Body parts affected
	L	L	L	M	L	Legs

With hunting, the fitness benefits depend on the sort of hunting you do. Lying patiently in a duck blind, you burn few calories and derive few fitness benefits. Stalking your prey on foot in the woods, you may cover many miles and burn many calories in the course of a day. An active chase may easily put your heart rate within the EBZ. But most people who enjoy hunting do not get many opportunities to achieve intensity with any regularity or frequency. So if you enjoy hunting but want to develop fitness, you would be wise to supplement this activity with a regular CRE program such as walking or jogging.

Interval circuit training (*see also* interval circuit training model program in Chapter 7)

Action	CRE	BC	MS	ME	F	Body parts affected
3 sets or 20 min.	H	H	H	H	M	Full body

Estimating calorie cost

| 3 sets or 20 min.: | **.062** × your weight × total minutes in action = approximate calories burned |

Jogging & running (*see also* walking /jogging/running model programs in Chapter 7)

Action	CRE	BC	MS	ME	F	Body parts affected
Jog, 5 to 7 mph; run, 8 to 10 mph	H	H	M	H	L	Legs, hips

Estimating calorie cost

Slow jog, 5 mph:	**.06** × your weight × total minutes in action = approximate calories burned
Fast jog, 7 mph:	**.092** × your weight × total minutes in action = approximate calories burned
Slow run, 8 mph:	**.104** × your weight × total minutes in action = approximate calories burned
Fast run, 10 mph:	**.129** × your weight × total minutes in action = approximate calories burned

Judo

Action	CRE	BC	MS	ME	F	Body parts affected
Moderate to vigorous	M	M	H	H	M	Full body

Estimating calorie cost

| Moderate: | **.049** × your weight × total minutes in action = approximate calories burned |
| Vigorous: | **.09** × your weight × total minutes in action = approximate calories burned |

Although the Japanese word *judo* means "gentle way," it is the name of a vigorous and popular form of martial art. Compared with some of the other combative sports, such as jiu-jitsu, judo is relatively mild and injury-free. This is probably because of the emphasis placed on proper supervision and instruction, especially for beginners.

Judo sessions are physically demanding and usually last for at least one hour. The sessions are capable of developing muscular strength and endurance as well as CRE. Flexibility does not receive any particular emphasis but may be a by-product of many of the exercises. The development of muscular strength and endurance is the result of tugging, pushing, pulling, and throwing a partner who offers resistance. CRE

187

development is the result of the intermittent bursts of high-intensity activity with a partner. This interaction with a partner is a type of interval training; when conducted for a long period of time it can benefit CRE.

Jumping (*see also* Track & field)

	CRE	BC	MS	ME	F	Body parts affected
	L	M	H	M	H	Legs, hips, trunk

Karate

Action	CRE	BC	MS	ME	F	Body parts affected
Moderate to vigorous	H	H	M	H	H	Full body

Estimating calorie cost

Moderate:	.049 × your weight × total minutes in action = approximate calories burned
Vigorous:	.09 × your weight × total minutes in action = approximate calories burned

The term karate has come to describe those martial arts characterized by a choreographed series of offensive and defensive maneuvers using the hands and feet to block, punch, and strike. Practicing karate three times a week for an hour at a time can be a good-to-excellent way to develop and maintain most of the fitness components.

Practice sessions are similar to dance classes. After a warm-up, the karate class performs the individual striking, punching, and blocking maneuvers. As the session progresses, these exercises are put together into combinations. A highly skilled individual can perform complex and vigorous combinations very rapidly. And they are usually continued for more than fifteen minutes. Such activity is capable of maintaining high levels of CRE.

Karate is equally effective in influencing body composition and can be useful for weight control. Many karate exercises require a full range of movement of the joints and can effectively develop flexibility as well as muscular endurance.

Lacrosse (*see also* Team sports)

Action	CRE	BC	MS	ME	F	Body parts affected
Moderate to vigorous	H	H	M	H	M	Legs, arms

Estimating calorie cost

Moderate:	**.052** × your weight × total minutes in action = approximate calories burned
Vigorous:	**.078** × your weight × total minutes in action = approximate calories burned

Modern dance (*see also* Dance)

Action	CRE	BC	MS	ME	F	Body parts affected
Floor warm-ups	L	M	L	H	H	Legs, hips, trunk, arms
Moving combinations	M	M	M	H	H	Legs, hips, trunk, arms

Estimating calorie cost

Moving combinations:	**.058** × your weight × total minutes in action = approximate calories burned

Orienteering (*see also* Hiking)

Action	CRE	BC	MS	ME	F	Body parts affected
Moderate to vigorous	H	H	M	H	L	Legs

Estimating calorie cost

Moderate:	**.049** × your weight × total minutes in action = approximate calories burned
Vigorous:	**.078** × your weight × total minutes in action = approximate calories burned

In competitive orienteering the object is to progress on foot over unfamiliar terrain (using only a detailed topographical map and a compass), make your way past a series of specified stations, and arrive first at the finish line. Contests are held over all types of terrain and they last for well over an hour. Participants need speed and endurance as they sprint, jog, climb, run, and walk through the course. Although the sport emphasizes problem-solving rather than athletic ability, high levels of CRE can help considerably. Train for this activity by hiking and jogging.

Outdoor fitness trails

Action	CRE	BC	MS	ME	F	Body parts affected
2.5-mile course	H	H	M	H	M	Full body

Estimating calorie cost

2.5-mile course:	**.06** × your weight × total minutes in action = approximate calories burned

189

The outdoor fitness trail is a novel idea that attempts to combine jogging (or walking) trails with a circuit of exercise stations. The activity originated in Switzerland in the late 1960s and is referred to as *parcours,* derived from a French term meaning "course" or "circuit." Fitness trails are receiving increased attention in the United States.

The *parcours* might be described as a "fitness playground" because of the jungle-gym nature of some of the exercise stations. Stations may number as many as twenty and vary in type as well as materials used. The total distance of the course also varies, depending on how far apart the stations are. The course may extend from about ¾ of a mile up to 2½ miles. Participants do sit-ups, pull-ups, or other exercises at each of the stations, then walk, jog, or run along the trail or path to the next station.

A typical course begins with a detailed map of the course and a description of how it is to be used. Directional signs guide you toward the stations. Each station has a sign that illustrates and explains how the exercise is to be performed and the number of repetitions of the exercise.

The outdoor fitness trail can serve as a good all-around fitness program for some people. The fact that it is outdoors offers a varied and attractive challenge that may be appealing. However, the potential fitness benefits of a particular trail will depend on whether the exercise stations are designed to develop muscular strength, endurance, and flexibility of all major muscle groups and whether the exerciser participates at an intensity high enough to maintain the heart rate within the EBZ for at least fifteen minutes and preferably longer.

Paddleball (*see also* Racquet, wall & net sports)

Action	CRE	BC	MS	ME	F	Body parts affected
Skilled, singles	H	H	M	H	M	Arms, shoulders, legs
Beginner, singles; all doubles	M	M	M	M	M	Arms, shoulders, legs

Estimating calorie cost

Beginner, singles; all doubles:	**.049** × your weight × total minutes in action = approximate calories burned
Skilled, singles:	**.078** × your weight × total minutes in action = approximate calories burned

Paddleball is played under the same conditions as handball, except that a wood paddle is used to strike a somewhat larger ball. The game is a bit faster than handball because the paddle increases the ball's velocity. However, the use of the paddle prevents putting spin on the ball—as is possible in handball—and eliminates the trick shots prominent in handball.

Paddle tennis (*see also* Racquet, wall & net sports)

Action	CRE	BC	MS	ME	F	Body parts affected
Skilled, singles	H	H	M	M	M	Legs, one side of upper body
Beginner, singles; all doubles	M	M	M	M	M	Legs, one side of upper body

Estimating calorie cost

Beginner, singles:	**.032** × your weight × total minutes in action = approximate calories burned
Skilled, doubles:	**.042** × your weight × total minutes in action = approximate calories burned
Skilled, singles:	**.055** × your weight × total minutes in action = approximate calories burned

Paddle tennis is just like tennis, except that it uses a short-handled wood paddle and a deadened tennis ball, and the court used is considerably smaller than a tennis court. It was originally devised as a playground game for children, but it has since become a full-blown competitive sport with tournaments and a national championship. It can be a fast-moving, exciting sport and a moderate source of improvement in all five fitness components.

Parallel bars (*see also* Gymnastics)

	CRE	BC	MS	ME	F	Body parts affected
	L	M	H	H	H	Arms, shoulders, trunk

Platform tennis (*see also* Racquet, wall & net sports)

Action	CRE	BC	MS	ME	F	Body parts affected
Skilled, singles	H	H	M	M	M	Full body
Beginner, singles; all doubles	M	M	M	M	M	Full body

Estimating calorie cost

Beginner, singles; all doubles:	**.049** × your weight × total minutes in action = approximate calories burned
Skilled, singles:	**.078** × your weight × total minutes in action = approximate calories burned

An offspring of paddle tennis, platform tennis was devised as an outdoor sport that could take place even when the tennis court was covered with snow. Platform tennis is played on a court constructed on a

191

wood platform, which is surrounded by a resilient wire fence originally designed to stop balls hit beyond the platform. The fence led to an additional rule that allows the ball to be hit off the wire fence if it has first bounced in the court. Platform tennis provides a good source of improvement in all five fitness components.

Pole vault (*see also* Track & field)

	CRE	BC	MS	ME	F	Body parts affected
	L	M	H	M	H	Arms, shoulders, legs, trunk

Racquetball (*see also* Racquet, wall & net sports)

Action	CRE	BC	MS	ME	F	Body parts affected
Skilled, singles	H	H	M	M	M	One side of body, trunk, legs
Beginner, singles; all doubles	M	M	M	M	M	One side of body, trunk, legs

Estimating calorie cost

Beginner, singles; all doubles: **.049** × your weight × total minutes in action = approximate calories burned

Skilled, singles: **.078** × your weight × total minutes in action = approximate calories burned

One of the fastest growing sports in the United States, racquetball is played on a court similar to the one used in four-wall handball. Racquetball is played with a short-handled racket, strung like a tennis racket. Courts are available at "Y" associations and colleges and at an ever-increasing number of private racquetball centers in cities and suburbs. A principal attraction of racquetball for many is its potential for developing CRE without requiring more than modest skill.

Racquet, wall & net sports (*see also* Badminton, Handball, Paddleball, Paddle tennis, Platform tennis, Racquetball, Squash, Table tennis, Tennis)

Badminton, tennis, paddle tennis, and platform tennis are all sports in which a ball or other missile is hit over a net with a racket or paddle. In racquetball, paddleball, and squash, players use rackets or paddles to hit a ball against one or more walls rather than over a net. In handball, the ball is played against one or more walls, but the fingers and palms of the hands are used to hit the ball. All these sports make similar fitness demands on their players, require similar skills, and produce comparable fitness benefits. They all demand good eye/hand coordination, the ability to start and stop quickly, and a stroking or swinging action of one or both arms. It's important to use an eye protector when playing any of these sports.

The potential of the racquet and wall sports for developing CRE depends on the duration, frequency, and intensity of your participation. Most of these games require at least thirty minutes to complete a match, so duration is simple to arrange. The intensity of the game can vary greatly, however, depending on the skill of the players. Singles play can easily bring the heart rate within the EBZ if the players are able to maintain a volley for a long enough time. But with players of limited ability, the active participation is so intermittent that it is difficult to achieve or sustain CRE.

Rock climbing

Action	CRE	BC	MS	ME	F	Body parts affected
Moderate to vigorous	M	M	H	H	H	Full body

Estimating calorie cost

Moderate to vigorous: **.033** × your weight × total minutes in action = approximate calories burned

Rock climbing involves ascending and descending steep cliffs or rock faces by means of hand and foot holds.

The activity requires—and will develop—muscular strength, muscular endurance, and flexibility. Pulling yourself up and stretching to reach the hand and foot holds contribute to these fitness components. *Belaying* (holding the safety ropes for your partner) and *rappelling* (rapid descent using a rope) require rope-handling skills and contribute to muscular strength and endurance. But rock climbing contributes moderately to CRE because the pace is generally slow and there are usually frequent rest periods.

If you are fit, you will find it easier to learn climbing skills. Fitness is also essential for the safety of all members of the climbing group. Climbing is a team effort: You are responsible for your safety and for the safety of others.

Because rock climbing is generally not practical as a regular activity, it should be a supplement to your regular fitness program.

Rope skipping (*see also* rope skipping model program in Chapter 7)

Action	CRE	BC	MS	ME	F	Body parts affected
70 to 100 turns per min.	H	H	M	H	L	Legs, forearms

Estimating calorie cost

70 turns per min.: **.071** × your weight × total minutes in action = approximate calories burned

80 turns per min.: **.079** × your weight × total minutes in action = approximate calories burned

90 turns per min.: **.087** × your weight × total minutes in action = approximate calories burned

100 turns per min.: **.095** × your weight × total minutes in action = approximate calories burned

Rowing

Action	CRE	BC	MS	ME	F	Body parts affected
Moderate to vigorous	H	H	H	H	H	Full body

Estimating calorie cost

Moderate: **.032** × your weight × total minutes in action = approximate calories burned

Vigorous: **.097** × your weight × total minutes in action = approximate calories burned

Competitive rowing—including *sweeps,* in which each crew member uses only one oar, and *sculls,* in which each person uses two—activates many major muscle groups. It is an excellent way to develop all the fitness components. (In a rowboat without a sliding seat, however, one gets little activity in the thigh muscles, thus limiting the CRE benefits derived from the sport.)

Practice sessions often involve one or two hours of high-intensity exercise, burning lots of calories and achieving CRE and body composition goals. Strenuous rowing, whether in an actual boat or a stationary rowing machine, also provides high levels of muscular strength, muscular endurance, and flexibility.

Recreational rowing in a traditional flat-bottomed rowboat can also be a good fitness activity if you row at adequate levels of intensity, duration, and frequency.

Royal Canadian Air Force (RCAF) program

Action	CRE	BC	MS	ME	F	Body parts affected
5BX & XBX	M	M	M	H	M	Full body

Estimating calorie cost

XBX, 5BX (Chart 1): **.055** × your weight × total minutes in action = approximate calories burned

XBX, 5BX (Chart 2): **.069** × your weight × total minutes in action = approximate calories burned

XBX, 5BX (Charts 3, 4): **.097** × your weight × total minutes in action = approximate calories burned

5BX (Charts 5, 6): **.111**× your weight × total minutes in action = approximate calories burned

This program was originally designed to meet the needs of Canadian Air Force personnel and their families. At first, it was available only through the Canadian government printing office. Later, a revised version was adopted for use by the United States Air Force. Still later, it became available as an inexpensive paperback book. The RCAF plan is primarily a calisthenic program of five basic exercises (5BX) for men and ten basic exercises (XBX) for women. By following detailed instructions and progressing from easy levels to age-specified goals, you begin with low intensities and a few repetitions and proceed from chart to chart until you reach a level appropriate for your age group. The recommended duration of the exercise session remains constant—eleven minutes to complete the 5BX and twelve minutes for the XBX. Common to both 5BX and XBX are toe touches, sit-ups, push-ups, and back extensions.

The exercises are well designed to improve muscular endurance and, to a lesser extent, muscular strength in the major muscle groups. Some of the exercises, particularly in the XBX program, could improve flexibility, especially if done through the full range of motion of the joints involved. But ideally, a well-rounded, balanced exercise plan should include more stretching. Similarly, some CRE training is provided by a three-minute stationary run in the XBX program, and by a six-minute stationary run (for which you may substitute in the 5BX program a one-mile run or a two-mile walk).

The exercises seem somewhat less than optimal as cardiorespiratory training. If you have been performing the 5BX or XBX regularly, or if you are considering undertaking either of these programs, precede your workout with the warm-up/cool-down in the stretching model program in Chapter 7. You should also balance out your program by increasing the stationary run or choosing some other form of CRE exercise. With such adaptations and supplements in mind, you can use the RCAF basic exercises as part of a sound fitness program.

Rugby (*see also* Team sports)

Action	CRE	BC	MS	ME	F	Body parts affected
Moderate to vigorous	H	H	M	H	M	Legs, trunk, arms, shoulders

195

Estimating calorie cost

Moderate:	$.052 \times$ your weight $\times$ total minutes in action = approximate calories burned
Vigorous:	$.097 \times$ your weight $\times$ total minutes in action = approximate calories burned

Sailing

	CRE	BC	MS	ME	F	Body parts affected
	L	L	L	M	L	Arms, shoulders, trunk

Whether you sail a small Sunfish-class boat for a few hours each weekend, or cruise for weeks on a thirty-foot sailboat, the fitness benefits of sailing are limited. Some improvement of muscular strength, muscular endurance, and flexibility may take place in the arms, shoulders, and the trunk as a result of regular sailing. But the activity is mainly recreational or competitive and should not be selected primarily to achieve fitness.

Scuba diving

Action	CRE	BC	MS	ME	F	Body parts affected
Moderate	M	M	M	H	M	Arms, shoulders, legs

Estimating calorie cost

Moderate:	$.045 \times$ your weight $\times$ total minutes in action = approximate calories burned

The word scuba is an acronym for Self-Contained Underwater Breathing Apparatus. This refers to the compressed air cylinders used by divers to stay underwater for extended periods of time. Air supply usually lasts about twenty minutes. The time spent underwater, however, can vary, depending on the diver's degree of exertion and how deep the diver swims. For scuba diving to provide fitness benefits, dives should be limited to thirty or thirty-five feet: The air supply will then last long enough to produce CRE effects.

Because scuba diving can be dangerous, it is important to seek instruction from certified instructors. Learning how to make this activity safe can also help make it effective.

Side horse (*see also* Gymnastics)

	CRE	BC	MS	ME	F	Body parts affected
	L	M	M	H	H	Arms, trunk

Skateboarding

Action	CRE	BC	MS	ME	F	Body parts affected
Moderate to vigorous	M	M	M	M	M	Legs

Estimating calorie cost

Moderate to vigorous: $.049 \times$ your weight $\times$ total minutes in action = approximate calories burned

    Enthusiastic skateboarders—usually youngsters between eight and fourteen years old—may spend hours perfecting the many styles and stunts required for organized competition or just plain fun. The activity resembles both skating and skiing, but it may not always provide CRE benefits because time may be spent coasting on a skateboard. Its primary value is in developing muscular endurance in the legs.

    Skateboarding, especially on streets and sidewalks, has its hazards. One should carefully consider the risk/benefit ratio before using skateboarding in a fitness program. Skateboarding without experience and training is, as one authority put it, "like jumping on a bar of soap." Wearing protective equipment such as a helmet, knee and elbow pads, wrist guards, and gloves may prevent injuries. It is also helpful if the skateboarder has some training in how to fall.

Skating/ice & roller

Action	CRE	BC	MS	ME	F	Body parts affected
Beginner to vigorous	M	M	M	H	M	Legs, hips

Estimating calorie cost

Beginner: $.032 \times$ your weight $\times$ total minutes in action = approximate calories burned

Moderate: $.049 \times$ your weight $\times$ total minutes in action = approximate calories burned

Vigorous: $.065 \times$ your weight $\times$ total minutes in action = approximate calories burned

    Most variants of ice and roller skating—including dance, disco, speed, and figure skating—require rhythmic large-muscle movements capable of developing CRE, improving body composition, and burning a great many calories over a long duration. To do this, of course, you must skate at high intensity for fifteen minutes or more at least three times a week.

    It may take some time to develop sufficient skill to use skating as a fitness exercise. But once you can skate well enough to enjoy the recrea-

197

tional and social aspects, you should be able to skate hard and fast enough to get your heart rate into the EBZ and achieve a CRE training effect. In addition to CRE, skating can improve flexibility, muscular endurance, and muscular strength, especially in the legs and hips.

Skiing/Alpine

Action	CRE	BC	MS	ME	F	Body parts affected
Continuous, intermediate to expert	M	M	H	H	M	Thighs, hips

Estimating calorie cost

Continuous, intermediate:	.039 × your weight × total minutes in action = approximate calories burned
Continuous, expert:	.078 × your weight × total minutes in action = approximate calories burned

Alpine, or downhill, skiing can develop moderate-to-high levels of fitness, depending on how well you ski and how fit you are to begin with. With moderate skill, skiing can supplement your regular fitness program, particularly in developing muscular strength and endurance in the thighs and hips.

If your ski runs exceed five to ten minutes, and if you can repeat them throughout the day—using the lift ride as a rest interval—you may even achieve some CRE benefits as well. Of course, you can modify your pace and select trails of varying difficulty to get the effect of interval training. High-intensity skiing requires muscular strength and endurance, as well as high CRE. Be sure to warm up and cool down adequately before and after each outing. However, because skiing is for most people only a weekend recreational activity, it should not be depended on as the mainstay of a fitness program.

Skin diving

Action	CRE	BC	MS	ME	F	Body parts affected
Moderate	M	M	M	H	M	Arms, shoulders, legs

Estimating calorie cost

Moderate:	.052 × your weight × total minutes in action = approximate calories burned

Skin diving uses no special oxygen supply. To view the scene below, swimmers float face down on the surface of the water. They use only a mask to cover their eyes and nose, a snorkel or long tube to let them breathe with their faces submerged, and fins attached to their feet to facilitate swimming through the water. Skin diving involves constant swimming near the surface, usually for thirty or more minutes at a time, so it is an effective CRE activity.

Snowshoeing

Action	CRE	BC	MS	ME	F	Body parts affected
2.5 mph	H	H	M	H	M	Legs, hips

Estimating calorie cost

2.5 mph: **.06** × your weight × total minutes in action = approximate calories burned

Snowshoes make it possible to walk on deep snow without sinking in all the way. You actually float on or near the surface, which permits you to move overland fairly efficiently even in deep snow. In snowy regions, snowshoeing provides avid hikers and walkers the opportunity to continue their outdoor activities year-round. Showshoeing is self-paced, and can provide moderate-to-high benefits in all five fitness components.

By using ski poles you can increase your stability, especially on hills, and also add arm and upper body exercise to the activity. The benefit you get from snowshoeing, of course, depends on your pace, the depth and softness of the snow, and the hilliness of the terrain.

Soccer (*see also* Team sports)

Action	CRE	BC	MS	ME	F	Body parts affected
Moderate to vigorous	H	H	M	H	M	Legs, trunk, neck

Estimating calorie cost

Moderate: **.052** × your weight × total minutes in action = approximate calories burned

Vigorous: **.097** × your weight × total minutes in action = approximate calories burned

Sprinting (*see also* Track & field)

	CRE	BC	MS	ME	F	Body parts affected
	L	M	H	M	M	Hips, legs

Squash (*see also* Racquet, wall & net sports)

Action	CRE	BC	MS	ME	F	Body parts affected
Skilled, singles	H	H	M	M	M	Arms, shoulders
Beginner, singles; all doubles	M	M	M	M		Arms, shoulders

Estimating calorie cost

Beginner, singles; all doubles:
.049 × your weight × total minutes in action = approximate calories burned

Skilled, singles:
.078 × your weight × total minutes in action = approximate calories burned

One of the fastest of all the racquet sports, squash (also known as squash racquets) is played on a small four-walled indoor court. Players must move fast, not only to get into position to return their opponent's shots, but also to keep out of each other's way in the limited playing area. Many people play squash because it provides an intense workout in a short space of time.

Stretching/warm-up & cool-down (*see also* stretching model program in Chapter 7)

	CRE	BC	MS	ME	F	Body parts affected
	L	L	L	L	H	Full body

Surfboarding

Action	CRE	BC	MS	ME	F	Body parts affected
Including swimming	M	M	M	M	M	Legs, upper body

Estimating calorie cost

Including swimming:
.078 × your weight × total minutes in action = approximate calories burned

Riding a surfboard over waves that move in toward a beach can be a vigorous activity capable of developing all five fitness components, if you continue the activity for extended periods of time on a regular basis. The major fitness benefits are derived before the actual surfing takes place—that is, while paddling the surfboard away from the shore toward the breaking waves. Paddling out, like swimming, works the muscles of the chest, arms, and shoulders. This may put surfers into the EBZ before they even begin to mount and balance themselves on their boards. While riding the board, skilled surfers often execute maneuvers requiring considerable athletic ability and fitness. They need excellent CRE and swimming skills to keep afloat in turbulent water for fifteen to thirty minutes.

Swimming (*see also* swimming model program in Chapter 7)

Action	CRE	BC	MS	ME	F	Body parts affected
20 to 55 yds. per min.	H	H	M	H	M	Arms, shoulders, chest

Estimating calorie cost

20 yds. per min.:   **.032** × your weight × total minutes in action = approximate calories burned

55 yds. per min.:   **.088** × your weight × total minutes in action = approximate calories burned

Synchronized swimming

Action	CRE	BC	MS	ME	F	Body parts affected
Moderate to vigorous	M	M	M	H	H	Full body

Estimating calorie cost

Moderate: **.032** × your weight × total minutes in action = approximate calories burned

Vigorous: **.052** × your weight × total minutes in action = approximate calories burned

Synchronized swimming (water ballet) is a group water activity performed in choreographed patterns in time to music. This combination of art and sport requires strong, proficient swimming skills, flexibility, and moderate-to-high levels of CRE and muscular endurance. Proficiency requires long hours of practice, usually as a member of a team or club representing a school or "Y." Practice sessions last at least an hour at a time and take place on a regular basis. This form of swimming is particularly helpful in developing flexibility and can produce training effects in CRE and muscular endurance equal to those of a swimming program.

Table tennis (*see also* Racquet, wall & net sports)

Action	CRE	BC	MS	ME	F	Body parts affected
Skilled	M	M	L	M	M	One side of body, wrist, arm

Estimating calorie cost

Skilled: **.045** × your weight × total minutes in action = approximate calories burned

The United States Table Tennis Association notes that the sport of table tennis, also known as Ping-Pong, is the second most popular participation sport in the world, surpassed only by soccer. Perhaps this is so because it's a game that allows people of any sex, age, size, and strength to play.

This game is a form of tennis played on a table. It can be played for fun—a leisurely, low-intensity game—or it can be quite vigorous, depending on the skills of the players. The fitness benefits, however, may be limited by a player's inability to perform at high skill levels or by lack of stiff competition.

Tai Chi Chuan

	CRE	BC	MS	ME	F	Body parts affected
	L	L	L	M	M	Full body

Tai Chi, as it is often called, is an ancient Chinese system of self-defense, based on a series of postures that are combined into routines. These are done slowly, with deep concentration, and with a flowing style. Tai Chi involves the whole body and can promote muscular endurance and flexibility. But it is of little use for developing CRE. If Tai Chi is the major element in your fitness program, you should incorporate into your program activities that promote CRE, body composition, and muscular strength.

Team handball (*see also* Team sports)

Action	CRE	BC	MS	ME	F	Body parts affected
Moderate to vigorous	H	H	M	H	M	Legs, arms

Estimating calorie cost

Moderate:	**.052** × your weight × total minutes in action = approximate calories burned
Vigorous:	**.078** × your weight × total minutes in action = approximate calories burned

Team sports (*see also* Basketball, Field hockey, Football/touch, Frisbee/ultimate, Hockey/ice & roller, Lacrosse, Rugby, Soccer, Team handball)

Of the running and skating team sports, basketball, field, ice, and roller hockey, football, lacrosse, rugby, soccer, team handball, and ultimate frisbee are highly competitive team games in which each team defends its goal against running and passing attacks from the opposing team. These games all require more or less continuous movement up, down, and across a field, court, or rink. So they demand and produce moderate-to-high levels of CRE and muscular endurance in the legs. The speed and continuity of the running or skating vary from sport to sport and from time to time within any game, with short bursts of speed followed by more leisurely runs (as in basketball or soccer) or with frequent shifting of personnel (as in the two-platoon system in football). Intensity also varies with the position you play. For example, the center-halfback on a soccer team is generally more active than a fullback, who may be relatively inactive if the team's offensive unit is dominating the game.

The major fitness benefits acquired from these sports come from practice sessions. In organized teams, these usually include warm-up exercises, jogging, and weight training, as well as fast moving drills and scrimmages. By improving your flexibility, muscular development, body composition, and CRE—both during the playing season and in the off-season—you can improve your performance, increase your protection against injury, and gain greater enjoyment on the playing field.

Tennis *(see also* Racquet, wall & net sports)

Action	CRE	BC	MS	ME	F	Body parts affected
Skilled, singles	H	H	M	M	M	One side of body, playing arm, shoulder, legs
Beginner, singles; all doubles	M	M	M	M	M	One side of body, playing arm, shoulder, legs

Estimating calorie cost

Beginner:	**.032** × your weight × total minutes in action = approximate calories burned
Skilled, doubles:	**.049** × your weight × total minutes in action = approximate calories burned
Skilled, singles:	**.071** × your weight × total minutes in action = approximate calories burned

Tennis requires good eye/hand coordination. It also demands speed and agility to get yourself into position to return the ball once your opponent has hit it to your side of the net. The intensity of play varies widely, depending on your skill and the skill of your opponent, the surface of the court, and especially on whether you are playing singles or doubles. In singles, you cover your entire side of the court, which could require a great deal of running with rapid starts and short stops. In doubles, partners take turns both serving and returning balls; they run less and hit fewer shots. You probably cannot rely on tennis to produce significant benefits in CRE or body composition, unless you are highly skilled and play frequently and for long durations. You can achieve a limited amount of muscular strength and endurance, especially in the legs and in the playing arm and shoulder.

The game requires a high degree of skill; lessons are recommended to get started.

Throwing/discus, hammer, javelin, shot put (*see also* Track & field)

CRE	BC	MS	ME	F	Body parts affected
L	M	H	H	M	Upper body, legs

Track & field (*see also* Jumping, Pole vault, Sprinting, Throwing)

Track and field is a general term covering competitive walking, running, jumping, and throwing events. The walking and running events are held on a track and may range from a short sprint to a six-mile run. Running events also include hurdle racing, which requires jumping over obstacles. Jumping events include the high jump, running broad jump, triple jump, and pole vault. Throwing, jumping, and short-distance sprinting events require power. Muscular strength, then, is an important fitness component in performing these events—hence the critical role of weight training in preparation for track and field events. Muscular endurance and flexibility are also necessary. The particular muscle groups to receive special attention depend on the event. The explosive events such as the jumps and sprints require anaerobic fitness (see page 54). CRE is the component most necessary for (and developed by) distance runners and walkers.

Track and field enthusiasts who are serious about their participation and adhere to any of the typical, currently accepted training regimens will usually have a high level of fitness for all components.

Trampoline (*see also* Gymnastics)

CRE	BC	MS	ME	F	Body parts affected
L	M	M	H	M	Legs, hips

Tumbling (*see also* Gymnastics)

CRE	BC	MS	ME	F	Body parts affected
L	M	H	H	H	Legs, hips, upper body

Twirling/baton

Action	CRE	BC	MS	ME	F	Body parts affected
Moderate to vigorous	M	M	M	H	H	Arms, shoulders

Estimating calorie cost

Continuous, for at least 15 min.:	**.049** × your weight × total minutes in action = approximate calories burned

Baton twirling is a highly specialized competitive sport as well as an entertainment feature of school and college athletic events. Performers sometimes execute spectacular maneuvers with the baton, often while marching but usually when stationary. Skilled participants are usually highly flexible and have good muscular endurance in the upper body. Continuous vigorous practice sessions can develop CRE, but baton twirling is primarily stationary. So beginners cannot rely on this activity for significant development of CRE.

Volleyball

Action	CRE	BC	MS	ME	F	Body parts affected
Moderate to vigorous	M	M	L	M	M	Arms, shoulders

Estimating calorie cost

Vigorous (skilled, competitive):	**.065** × your weight × total minutes in action = approximate calories burned

The fitness benefits of volleyball can range from minimal to considerable, depending on the skills of the players and the conditions under which the game is played. Most of us are familiar with beach or backyard volleyball, involving people of all ages, sexes, and skills. The games can be fun but they are actually of little fitness value. Competitive volleyball is a different story. Played at the high school, intercollegiate, amateur, and even Olympic levels, it has grown increasingly popular in recent years. At these levels, volleyball includes vigorous leaping, spiking, blocking, and diving; and it can develop CRE as well as muscular endurance and flexibility. These fitness benefits are particularly available to members of an established team that practices regularly for one to two hours each session.

Walking (*see also* walking/jogging/running model programs in Chapter 7)

Action	CRE	BC	MS	ME	F	Body parts affected
Slow to fast walk, 2.5 to 4.5 mph	H	H	L	H	L	Hips, legs

Estimating calorie cost

Moderate, 3.5 mph: $.029 \times$ your weight $\times$ total minutes in action = approximate calories burned

Fast, 4.5 mph: $.048 \times$ your weight $\times$ total minutes in action = approximate calories burned

Water polo

Action	CRE	BC	MS	ME	F	Body parts affected
Vigorous	H	H	M	H	M	Arms, shoulders, legs

Estimating calorie cost

Vigorous: $.078 \times$ your weight $\times$ total minutes in action = approximate calories burned

Water polo, a game like field hockey or football but played in a lake or swimming pool, is a rough contact sport. Swimmers score points by shooting a ball slightly smaller than a basketball into a net in the pool. Players must be fast and skillful swimmers, with high levels of muscular endurance and CRE. They must be able to change swimming direction without losing time or momentum, and with or without the ball. Training for and participation in water polo can develop all five fitness components.

Waterskiing

Action	CRE	BC	MS	ME	F	Body parts affected
Moderate to vigorous	M	M	M	H	M	Arms, thighs

Estimating calorie cost

Moderate: $.039 \times$ your weight $\times$ total minutes in action = approximate calories burned

Vigorous: $.055 \times$ your weight $\times$ total minutes in action = approximate calories burned

Waterskiing requires and can develop muscular endurance of the arms and thighs. Its value for CRE depends on whether the skier has adequate skill and muscular endurance to sustain fifteen minutes of continuous waterskiing. If you water-ski three or four times a week and can do intermediate and advanced skiing maneuvers, waterskiing can serve as a good fitness activity.

Weight training (*see also* weight training model program in Chapter 7)

	CRE	BC	MS	ME	F	Body parts affected
	L	M	H	H	H	Full body

Wrestling

Action	CRE	BC	MS	ME	F	Body parts affected
Moderate to vigorous	H	H	H	H	H	Full body

Estimating calorie cost

Moderate: **.065** × your weight × total minutes in action = approximate calories burned

Vigorous, competitive: **.094** × your weight × total minutes in action = approximate calories burned

A demanding sport, wrestling requires a high level of conditioning in each of the fitness components. Practice sessions last at least an hour. Typically, they include a warm-up period with considerable stretching, followed by a long session of drill on the many offensive and defensive maneuvers. These are followed by sparring matches, organized by weight classification. The vigorous activity can promote muscular endurance as well as CRE. The resistance offered by opponents improves muscular strength and provides the necessary twisting and turning to develop flexibility.

Yoga

	CRE	BC	MS	ME	F	Body parts affected
	L	L	L	M	H	Full body

As it is practiced most frequently in the United States today, yoga is primarily the method of Hatha yoga, the most physical of the traditional Hindu systems of philosophy that attempt to unite the mind and body in a tranquil union. In a typical Hatha yoga session, people go through a series of *asanas,* that is, slow rhythmic movements that gently ease the body into comfortably stretched positions that are held without motion for varying lengths of time. The *asanas* are performed in a balanced sequence so that participants systematically put all joints and muscle groups through a full range of motion. Yoga is the most effective way to achieve and maintain flexibility. Some muscular endurance may also accrue. While yoga is of minimal value for CRE, body composition, and muscular strength, it may be helpful for people with low levels of muscular development who wish to get started in a fitness program.

Many joggers, runners, cyclists, and others whose primary exercise tends to tighten specific muscle groups have begun to recognize the value of yoga to improve flexibility and, in many cases, to help them remain free of injury.

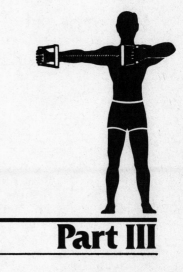

Part III

CHAPTER

9

Commercial and Institutional Fitness Facilities

Choosing a fitness facility can be a complicated exercise in itself. There is a multitude of spas, centers, and programs based on every kind of physical fitness "system." There is the "no-sweat" path to fitness offered by some health clubs and so-called figure salons that focus on yoga-type stretching movements. Other facilities pattern their exercise programs on non-strenuous dance exercise or gymnastic skills. Many provide sophisticated weight training equipment and emphasize muscular development. Still others offer a range of activities wide enough to include medically supervised programs to develop cardiorespiratory fitness.

Facilities with a balanced program emphasize instruction geared to the development of all five of the fitness components: cardiorespiratory endurance (CRE), body composition, muscular strength, muscular endurance, and flexibility. Some supply no-nonsense, balanced fitness programs that can get you in and out without wasting your time. Other programs, such as those conducted by community recreation departments, stress fun and recreation, with physical fitness treated almost like a side effect. Some combination racquet-and-health clubs and spas offer a variety of approaches. In addition, some large corporations provide employees with in-house fitness facilities.

The image of the gymnasium as a stark, sweat-scented space containing shabby and half-broken exercise equipment seems to be on the way out. The new image is one of attractive, shiny, sophisticated equipment, carpeted floors, mirrored walls, and other decorator-look appointments. Unfortunately, this classy image is sometimes marred by reports of shoddy business practices.

As *Consumer Reports* noted in August 1978: "There are more than 3,000 health spas around the nation, ranging from small exercise rooms and reducing salons to multimillion-dollar facilities with gymnasiums, swimming pools, running tracks, saunas, whirlpools, and the like. Some

210

spas are clearly consumer-oriented attempts to promote physical fitness, with such fair business practices as pro rata refunds at any time. Others are barely one step ahead of the nearest district attorney.... If the volume of complaints flowing into consumer agencies is any indication, many health-spa customers are concluding that the only thing getting trimmed is their wallet."

A number of readers of *Consumer Reports* have described for us some of the reasons they joined health spas or gyms or other organized programs.

■ "I was most successful with my exercise program when I scheduled it for a particular day and time every week. I didn't spend a lot of money, but knowing I was really wasting money I had spent if I didn't go to the activity gave me that extra push."

■ "I like class/group exercise. Peer pressure and sociability provide motivation after an exhausting day at work."

■ "I think that having a set time of the week and a special time of the day to do...exercises, and especially having someone to do them with, really helps."

Choosing a facility

If you prefer an organized program—the kind offered by commercial fitness centers or by institutions— you should base your selection of one on answers to these questions.

Is the cost of membership within your means, and the contract, if any, in your best interests? If the cost of joining an organized exercise facility is going to be a drain on your pocketbook, don't join. Review the principles of exercise outlined in Chapter 2 of this book. And check the model programs in Chapter 7 and the sports and activities in Chapter 8. Thus armed, you should be able to set up your own exercise program, which would certainly be less costly.

If cost is not a factor, shop around for the best deal but measure the price against what you get in return. Be sure to find out about any extra charges for the use of courts or other special facilities or services. Another policy that affects cost is whether you are credited for enforced absences because of illness or vacation. Be suspicious of high-pressure selling and long-term contracts. Don't sign a contract until all your questions are answered.

Does the facility request appropriate medical information and, if necessary, medical clearance? Some facilities require an exercise stress test and medical clearance after which they may conduct a fitness evaluation (including a skinfold measurement to assess body fat). This information is then used to design an individualized program.

If the facility you're considering does not require medical clearance

211

and other pertinent information, follow the guidelines outlined in Chapter 1. Whether you're asked or not, tell the staff about any medical problems you may have.

Is the staff qualified to provide exercise instruction? If you want the best in fitness counseling, then you must be certain that those doing the counseling are fully qualified. Since qualified professionals receive salaries commensurate with their credentials, you should expect to pay more to a facility with such a staff. (Exceptions are nonprofit organizations such as the various "Y" associations, community centers, and recreation programs, and college or university programs.)

If none of the facilities you must choose among has a fully qualified staff but otherwise meets your needs, then you can still manage if you take on the responsibility of designing your exercise program yourself by applying the principles of exercise presented in Chapter 2.

Does the facility offer opportunities for developing all five of the fitness components? If you want a balanced program, you'll need either equipment or techniques that stress development of the cardiorespiratory and muscular systems. If a facility lacks such options as rowing machines, stationary bicycles, treadmills, or running space, then you may have difficulty in improving CRE. If resistance equipment is lacking, then you should not expect to develop your muscular strength and endurance to any great extent.

Exercise programs that stress "no sweat" and simple stretching movements can develop no more than flexibility. If you enjoy such limited programs, by all means participate. But be aware that you won't have a balanced program or one that will develop CRE. Even if the facility you plan to join does not have the resources to contribute to all five of the fitness components, it may have a professional staff that knows how to compensate for the gap. With circuit training or interval training, and such exercises as aerobic dance, the lack of some equipment may be overcome.

Is the equipment sufficient so that waiting is unnecessary, even at peak hours? An attractively decorated gym with shiny new equipment is all too often accepted as proof that the facility is adequately equipped. The only way to be certain, however, is to visit during peak hours. If people have to wait for a turn at the exercise equipment at those times, then the gym is overcrowded (or underequipped).

Some types of exercise programs require at least a minimum time at certain exercises (a stationary bicycle, for example) or performance of a circuit or interval training within specified target times. The value of such exercise programs may be impaired if you cannot get access to the equipment for sufficient time or at the appropriate time.

Are time limitations imposed? Limited access is sometimes the result of overcrowding. But other time restrictions are sometimes built into the rules—alternate days for men and women, or "men only" and "women only" during certain hours, for instance. The times you can then attend may not fit in with your plans, so be sure to find out when the facility will be available to you before you commit yourself.

Is there a system for evaluating your progress? A system for recording your progress is a necessity to provide progressive overload. Some programs provide individualized exercise cards that the participant uses during each visit. The system is more effective if a qualified instructor reviews the card on a regular basis so that adjustments in your program can be made as needed. If the facility does not provide progress cards but it meets your needs in other ways, be sure to set up your own record-keeping system (see Chapter 6).

Are enough instructors available to give you help when you need it? If one of your reasons for considering a commercial or institutional facility is to receive guidance in achieving your fitness goals, then be sure that enough qualified instructors are available. Facilities can work differently: Some require you to make an appointment for assistance; others have instructors who circulate and offer suggestions on the spot or who check your progress card at regular intervals and offer advice. Whatever the system, be certain that you understand it and can make full use of it. The system must be one that you will be comfortable with if it is to be effective for you.

Is the location convenient? In addition to finding a facility that's open on the days and during the hours best suited to your schedule, it's important to choose one that is conveniently located. If you can find time during the day for exercise, choose a facility that's close to where you work. Or if early mornings or evenings are best, then try to find a facility close to your home or at a handy point between your home and your job.

If you work for a corporation that sponsors a fitness program, make use of it. Employee programs are usually adjuncts of the company's medical department. These programs are usually supervised by qualified professionals (physical educators with knowledge or experience in exercise physiology).

Are there enough activities to hold your interest over a period of time? Some exercisers are so well disciplined that they can take regular exercise as though it were a measured dose of medicine. If you are one of these, then you should choose a facility that can provide a program consistent with the principles of exercise outlined in Chapter 2. If, however, you expect enjoyment along with your exercise, be certain that the available

213

activities are the kind you like. If you like to try new sports and exercises, select a facility with a wide variety of activities to choose from. If your family is to be involved in the program, then the scope of choices may have to be even broader.

Can the facility design a program for your special medical needs, if any?
A question to be resolved before you join an exercise facility is whether it can provide the necessary exercises you require should you have a particular health problem. There are specialized exercise programs, for instance, for cardiac rehabilitation, orthopedic problems, and other special physical needs. Most of these programs are associated with educational institutions, hospitals, medical centers, and the various "Y" associations. An occasional private club may also offer these special services.

10

Exercise and Youngsters, Women, and Older People

Of the more than a thousand readers of *Consumer Reports* who wrote to describe their experiences with exercise (or nonexercise), many asked specific questions about physical activity in childhood and during school years, and about exercise for women and older people. This chapter responds to some of these questions and concerns.

At what age should children begin to exercise? Actually children are, in effect, exercising when they are born. Most authorities on child development agree that kicking, grasping, reaching, crawling, turning over, and even crying—in short, all an infant's gross motor activities in the first few months of life—are crucial not only for healthy physical development but also because they lay the sensorimotor foundations of intellectual development as well. Cribs, playpens, and other equipment should permit safe, comfortable, relatively unrestricted movement.

During the preschool years, most toddlers need no prodding to walk, run, jump, climb, kick, throw, dig, lift, push, and pull—alone and with others. Mastery of such activities provides children with a sense of accomplishment, peer acceptance, and a foundation for later success in sports and games.

What are the physiological benefits of exercise for children? The benefits of cardiorespiratory endurance (CRE) training are apparent even in young children. Ten-year-olds who regularly train for age-group running competition, for example, tend to be taller, weigh less, and have greater aerobic capacity and lower percentages of body fat than youngsters who do not exercise regularly. This should not be surprising because from childhood on those who engage in regular physical activity, based on the principles of exercise described in Chapter 2, will raise their fitness levels above those who remain inactive.

Can strenuous training damage the heart of a growing child? No. There is no evidence that vigorous exercise will damage a healthy heart.

What can parents do to protect children from heart disease? In general, parents should encourage their children to do what adults are advised to do, and guard against the same risks that adults are advised to avoid. Children should exercise to cut down on the chance of obesity. The best forms of exercise for this purpose are bicycling, hiking, jogging, skating, cross-country skiing, and swimming. Competitive and team sports can also help if they require CRE. Sports such as basketball, hockey, soccer, and track and field are among those that seem to have the greatest appeal for boys and girls.

At what age can children start weight training? With proper safeguards, weight training can start whenever a child shows interest in the activity (see page 89). Particular attention should be paid to exercising both sides of the body equally and to developing strength and endurance in both flexor and extensor muscle groups in all the limbs. Properly done, weight training can protect against injury to the bones and joints of youngsters who are involved in active competitive sports. (See weight training model program in Chapter 7.)

Is Osgood-Schlatter disease, so common in children, a serious threat to exercise? The condition is painful but not usually dangerous. It gets better by itself in a few weeks or months. The disease is marked by pain, swelling, and tenderness just below one or both knees, at the point where the kneecap ligament joins the bone of the lower leg. It occurs in girls between the ages of eight and thirteen and, more often, in boys between ten and fifteen. A diagnosis of the disease should be considered tentative until confirmed by X rays. The best treatment is rest; several months may be needed. Recovery is usually complete and uneventful and physical activity can be resumed.

Doesn't a youngster with a fractured leg need exercise while the leg is in a cast? Yes, indeed. A youngster—or for that matter, an adult—who remains completely inactive while a fracture heals will decline rapidly in general fitness. When the cast comes off, these people have a double problem: The atrophied leg needs reconditioning—and so does the rest of the body. To guard against this, young fracture patients should learn to use crutches properly and use them as much as possible. Parents should chauffeur their children only when distance offers no alternative. Check with the school physical education department about an individualized fitness program to keep the student in shape without endangering the injured limb. If necessary, parents can help their young invalids design an exercise program based on the exercises in the Glossary of Exercises.

Exercises done while seated or lying down are most appropriate. After the cast comes off, the injured leg will return to normal much more readily if the patient has been regularly exercising other parts of the body, including the cardiorespiratory system, during the recovery period.

Are sports such as baseball, football, and hockey dangerous for growing children? The most dangerous of sports injuries in the young has to do with fractures of the growth regions of the long bones. These regions, called epiphyses, are attached but not solidly united to the main shaft of the bone until growth is completed. Injuries to the epiphyses are relatively infrequent, and when they do occur, the possibility of growth disturbance is even less frequent. Occasionally, an injury to the epiphyses does result in permanent damage to the limb. Most physicians and parents agree, however, that the benefits of participating in organized sports far outweigh the risk.

Should parents encourage their children to participate in competitive sports? Yes and no. Body type should be considered when deciding about such body-contact sports as hockey, football, or basketball. The obese child, or the tall gangly youngster with poor muscular development is particularly susceptible to injury. Such youngsters should probably wait until muscular development is more complete. Fitness programs can condition them for competition at a later time.

Another point to consider is how the competitive sports program is organized. If there is competent medical and educational supervision of practice and play, the benefits of competitive sports are increased and the hazards diminished.

Another consideration is the extent to which the sport contributes to fitness. Cardiorespiratory fitness does not automatically result from participation in competitive athletics. Unfortunately, most ball sports geared to eight- to nine-year-olds do not require high levels of intensity to improve CRE. The racquet sports are too difficult for many young children; it takes considerable time before they can acquire enough skill to turn frustration into pleasure or to keep the activity in the exercise benefit zone (EBZ, see pages 62–66) long enough to be effective for CRE. Running, ice and roller skating, swimming, or even many of the early childhood tag-and-chase games provide satisfactory conditioning for children at varying ages.

How can parents evaluate a competitive sports program for health and safety factors? A good athletic program for young people should provide (1) adequate conditioning, (2) intelligent instruction and coaching, (3) the best possible equipment and facilities, (4) competent officiating, and (5) expert medical care. The young participants, of course, should be physically qualified for the sport and about equal in growth and development.

217

Coaches should be aware of the principles of fitness training, and they should work with all members of their teams to achieve high levels of conditioning. The tendency in community programs, unfortunately, is for the least skilled players to be left sitting on the bench most of the time while the youngsters with the greatest skill and talent get to play and practice. The less skillful players who need the most training, practice, and attention from the coaching staff are often left to shift for themselves. They get bored or discouraged and ultimately quit.

What should parents look for in a school's physical education program? A physical education program should provide opportunities for students to develop and maintain fitness, to learn and practice movement skills, and to profit from the social and emotional experience of play, teamwork, and competition. The classes should help young people develop the motor skills needed for sports and games, with particular emphasis on those most likely to provide fitness in adult life. How well the classes meet these goals depends on many things from the competence of the teachers to the instructional time available for each student. If class time for physical education is limited, students may not have an adequate opportunity to develop fitness.

Too many school programs focus on the gifted athletes—those who make the varsity teams—and neglect those students who need training the most. Handicapped children require programs specially designed to their physical and emotional needs. Also, children with low performance levels in any of the fitness components need specially designed programs to work on their deficiencies, with periodic testing to help monitor progress.

For all children (as for adults), muscular strength and endurance and flexibility can be developed and maintained in sessions as short as fifteen minutes, three times per week. Cardiorespiratory fitness and changes in body composition may be achieved in activities with high CRE potential. To affect body composition, however, an exercise session must last at least thirty minutes and should occur more than three times a week.

In some elementary schools, the physical education program includes "movement education." Does this develop physical fitness? It can. Movement education is a relatively new approach to physical education in the primary grades. It's based on the idea that youngsters need instruction and encouragement in developing basic motor skills, which develop in different ways in each child. In movement classes, children practice a wide variety of simple activities, such as running, jumping, skipping, balancing, catching, and throwing. These movements are fundamental to sports, games, dance, and other activities that become important to them as they grow older. The classes can make a substantial contribution to the youngsters' muscular and cardiorespiratory endurance. It is not unusual

218

to observe students in these classes performing twenty to thirty minutes of continuous activity strenuous enough to keep their heart rate well within their EBZ. Thus movement education is a good way for elementary schools to improve students' motor skills (agility, balance, coordination, power, reaction time, and speed) without neglecting CRE or the other fitness components.

What can schools do for overweight or obese children? Some schools provide special programs for overweight youngsters in which small groups meet five times per week with specially trained teachers. Class time (usually forty-five minutes) is devoted to active team sports, in which the children are kept moving for almost the entire session. It is helpful when these classes are supplemented by discussions of good eating habits, encouragement of after-school activity, and elimination of junk foods from the school cafeteria. Preliminary results from this kind of program have been encouraging.

Is time spent in physical education classes on discussion, texts, and even homework worthwhile? The intellectual exploration of fitness concepts may seem less important than the physical pursuit of fitness, but in the long run it can help students make informed decisions about their future exercise programs. It is as important to understand the how and why of physical activity as it is to be able to perform that activity. Class time used to teach the fundamentals for a lifetime of physical fitness is certainly not misspent.

What accounts for the differences in fitness and athletic ability between men and women? It is obvious that the best male athletes run, swim, jump, and throw faster, higher, and farther than the best female athletes. Whether these differences in performance derive chiefly from biological superiority or are primarily the result of cultural differences and societal attitudes or both is open to debate. If you compare the strength, endurance, and body composition of large groups of male and female athletes, there are few actual differences between the fittest females and the fittest males. The range of difference is certainly wider within either sex than between the sexes.

Of course, there are inescapable biological differences between the sexes. Since girls tend to develop and mature more quickly than boys, they often outperform boys during childhood and adolescence. Once past adolescence, however, males tend to have a number of physical advantages over females. Males are generally taller, heavier, stronger, and faster. Their heart size and lung surface are usually greater and their hemoglobin levels are higher, hence their cardiac output and aerobic capacity are greater and their heart rate is generally slower. Their muscle mass is greater, so they are capable of generating more power. They have less body fat to supply with oxygen, so their cardiorespiratory system can deliver it more efficiently to the working muscles. Lastly, their shoulders are usually wider and their extremities longer in relation to trunk size, so they have a longer reach and stride than females. All of these generalizations, however, are based on averages: Within the normal physical ranges, there is, of course, a large area of overlap in which individual females outperform individual males.

There is also a marked difference in the way most families, schools, and communities encourage athletic participation for boys and girls from the earliest ages. High-caliber female performance has been limited by the amount of coaching time and effort women get, and by the quality and quantity of the facilities provided for them. Since both physical fitness and motor skills improve with conditioning, instruction, and practice, most women have been at a distinct disadvantage almost from birth when compared with men. Such circumstances, and the attitudes that bring them about, have been changing in American society. Many parents are now equally comfortable giving their daughters sports equipment as they are giving them dolls or housekeeping equipment. And schools receiving government funds are required to provide equal opportunity to girls and boys in physical education classes and in after-school programs.

Can vigorous activity cause iron deficiency in women? No. There is no evidence that exercise, no matter how vigorous, will deplete iron stores or cause iron-deficiency anemia in women who have an adequate diet.

Iron is required for the formation of hemoglobin, the substance in blood that transports oxygen to the cells. Dietary iron is found in meats (especially liver), fish, green leafy vegetables (not just spinach), beans, dried fruits, and whole wheat. It is more readily absorbed, however, from meats and fish than from vegetables and fruits. The body stores iron in the liver, spleen, and bone marrow. When blood is lost from the body and dietary intake is insufficient, then iron reserves become depleted and the production of red blood cells is impaired. The result is iron-deficiency anemia—the red cells become smaller, paler, and fewer than normal. With insufficient hemoglobin, the delivery of oxygen to the tissues becomes less efficient, and this, of course, decreases aerobic capacity and CRE.

Iron-deficiency anemia can place severe limits on a woman's fitness program. If your hemoglobin level is less than normal, you may tire easily and have great difficulty engaging in even mild exercise. No matter how regularly you work out, you may not be able to achieve the training effects you are striving for. If you find yourself in this sort of predicament, you should consult a physician.

Are contact sports such as hockey and soccer more dangerous for females? No. Thus far it has not been shown that females are physiologically more vulnerable to injury than males who already participate in contact sports. It is well known that there is a relatively high injury rate among males who engage in certain sports. The data for females, however, are limited. One study indicated that college women in sports such as basketball, field hockey, and lacrosse experience more injuries than women who play less hazardous sports such as tennis or softball. But these injuries are generally the same sprained ankles and knee injuries that are common among males. Injuries to breasts were the least common injuries. It appears that if women are given the same level of coaching, training, equipment, and practice time as men receive, they are no more likely to be injured in contact sports than men.

Is it all right to continue a vigorous exercise program while menstruating? Yes. No harm can come of it. The experience of menstruation varies greatly. For some women, it is accompanied by symptoms such as headache, backache, abdominal pain, and leg cramps. These symptoms should not create the impression that menstruation is a form of illness and that, as such, it is not advisable to exercise at that time. However, some women may not feel like exercising during menstruation, or at least during the first day or two when the menstrual discharge is usually heaviest and the discomfort, if any, is greatest. Many women experience little or no discomfort and thus rarely need to alter their exercise programs. Still others find that exercise helps reduce painful or uncomfortable symptoms of menstruation. In any case, there is no evidence that exercise during menstruation is unhealthy, or that there is any unfavorable effect on the way women athletes perform if they compete during menstruation.

Women should exercise at whatever intensity and duration they feel comfortable with during their menstrual periods. The key is to listen to your body: It's an individual decision.

Is it safe to go swimming while menstruating? Yes. There is no evidence that either the exertion of swimming or the submersion in water (cold or heated) can harm a menstruating female.

Is it true that exercise can cause cessation of menstrual cycles? No. However, most women who engage in high-CRE activities, such as long-distance running or cross-country skiing, have very low percentages of body fat, often as low as 10 percent. There appears to be a relationship between a woman's percentage of body fat and ovulation and menstruation. Thus women who are severely underweight or malnourished and women who go on crash diets or who for some other reason experience a rapid loss of weight may cease to ovulate and menstruate. Stress may also be a factor among athletes who experience this condition (called amenorrhea). They have the psychological stress of high-level competition as well as the physiological stresses imposed by rigorous training and significant weight loss. Once the stress is relieved—for example, if the woman regains the lost weight or reduces her level of training—normal menstrual cycles usually resume. (Because there are other causes of amenorrhea, a woman should not assume that lack of periods is caused by exercise. An examination by a gynecologist would be prudent.)

Can exercise such as jogging or rope skipping cause a woman's breasts to stretch or sag? Exercise does not cause sagging or stretching of the breasts. Aging or multiple pregnancies are more likely causes. However, some women athletes report soreness and tenderness of the breasts. Some studies have suggested that a well-fitted bra can reduce such discomfort. Whether a woman wears a bra during exercise is a matter of personal comfort and preference, often dependent on the size of the breasts.

Will running enlarge a woman's calves and thighs? Probably not. Like weight training, running need not develop bulky leg muscles. Women usually find that running burns up enough calories to reduce body fat, some of which may come off the hips and thighs. Running may also cause the leg muscles to become firmer and less flabby, without necessarily becoming larger.

Should pregnant women avoid exercise? No. Although some think otherwise, there is no evidence to suggest that exercise is detrimental for healthy pregnant women. Exercise won't deprive the fetus of needed energy or nourishment, nor will vigorous activity injure the fetus or cause a miscarriage. The fetus is well protected by the fluid in the amniotic sac and the supply of oxygen and nutrients through the placenta is not blocked by any activity the mother may engage in.

Indeed, there are many positive advantages of exercise in pregnancy. Increasing or maintaining CRE should help a pregnant woman feel better and have more energy than she might otherwise have. Exercises that improve body composition can help control excessive weight gain during pregnancy. And exercises to increase muscular strength and endurance, especially of the abdominal muscles and the muscles of the lower back and pelvic floor, can help a pregnant woman support the weight of the growing fetus comfortably, avoid back pain, and prepare for the muscular activity of labor. Exercises to increase or maintain flexibility are useful in overcoming some of the awkwardness and discomfort of the last trimester, as well as in preparing the body for labor and delivery. Finally, exercise in pregnancy—as in other stages of life—may improve self-esteem, help prevent insomnia, constipation, low-back pain, and leg cramps.

Engaging in competitive sports can present some problems for a pregnant woman. Most athletes stop competing when pregnancy causes their performance levels to drop. Usually by the third trimester, a woman's motor skills (such as agility, balance, and speed) would be affected. But pregnancy is no reason to let overall fitness decline. Quite the contrary. You may have to shift to more comfortable activities, but unless your physician advises inactivity, you should be able to stay in condition—or even improve your fitness—during pregnancy.

It is wise to consult your obstetrician before you *increase* your activities during pregnancy. And you should follow the basic fitness training principles outlined in Chapter 2. (See also Chapter 11, pages 236–241.)

How soon after giving birth can a woman resume exercising? That depends, of course, on the exercise. A woman should not undertake a full range of activity or rigorous exercise until about four to six weeks after giving birth. However, many obstetricians recommend specific exercises that can begin almost immediately following delivery. Exercises for the stretched abdominal muscles can be very helpful in improving muscle strength after childbirth. But avoid movements that stretch or strain the abdominal or pelvic floor muscles.

When you resume an exercise program (as you would when starting a new one), begin slowly and add gradually to the intensity and duration of your workouts. As your body gains strength, you should be able to resume all your usual activities. By six months after delivery, you should be able to exercise without any limitations.

Is vigorous exercise all right for a woman who is breastfeeding? Yes. Exercise for which a woman has gradually conditioned herself should not interfere with lactation.

Should people begin to take it easy when they retire? No. Retiring from a job doesn't mean you have to retire from everything else. If you have enjoyed certain physical activities throughout your life and are in good health, there is no reason to discontinue them.

Can a retired person begin exercising for the first time? Yes. Many people begin regular exercise for the first time after reaching retirement age. No matter what your age, you must listen to your body. If, for instance, jogging a mile feels like too much, then be satisfied with a half mile. Or break the mile up, doing half in the morning and half at night. Or walk instead of jog, or try another form of activity entirely, such as swimming or biking. There is no need to feel that you must jog just because it seems to be such a popular form of CRE training.

If people weigh the same at age sixty-five as they did in college, doesn't that mean they have remained physically fit? Not necessarily. Body weight is not a reliable measure of fitness. As explained in Chapters 1 and

4, body weight does not always accurately reflect whether you are fat. (Your weight could seem to be on the high side because you are heavily muscled, for example.) And even if you have maintained favorable body composition since your college days, you may still be less than fit in the other four fitness components. To find out how fit you are, assess your CRE, muscular strength, muscular endurance, and flexibility, as well as your body composition, following the suggestions in Chapter 1.

Does the ratio of fat to muscle necessarily increase as a person ages? In general, the percentage of body fat does increase with advancing age. But it is impossible to know how much of this increase is due to the aging process and how much is due to atrophy of muscle tissue because of declining activity. It is true that people who continue to exercise into and beyond middle age do maintain leaner bodies than do sedentary people. But since even active people gain some fat as they grow older, it would be wise to cut back on calories. As activity levels decline, older people should adjust caloric intake to caloric output.

Is sixty-five too late to start weight training? No. People in their sixties or seventies probably cannot accomplish quite as much improvement in muscular strength and endurance or increase the size of their muscles quite as much as people at younger ages. But it is certainly worthwhile to work on muscular fitness no matter what your age. Of course, you should be careful to begin with very low resistance and to add overload gradually. And it would be wise to check with your physician first.

Is there a specific age when the body begins to go downhill? Some physiological functions peak at the age of twenty, while others peak at thirty. It is difficult to know whether any physical decline is due to the effects of aging or whether it has to do with how inactive a person is. One thing is fairly clear, however: Older athletes do seem able to delay the aging process better than do sedentary people. Regular exercise that prevents the accumulation of excess fat and maintains high cardiorespiratory function can certainly help to protect a person from the so-called degenerative diseases of aging.

Is there an age beyond which training effects should no longer be expected? No. Age is no deterrent to the improvement of physical fitness. Although it's best to begin exercising young and continue throughout life, it is certainly better to begin exercising late than not at all. A sound, regular exercise program begun late in life will not regain for you the level of fitness you may have had in your youth. Nor should you expect to achieve training benefits as rapidly as a younger person might. However, there is no question that your fitness levels will improve if you follow a sensible program.

What precautions should older people take before beginning an exercise program? Before you undertake any new form of exercise, follow the advice in Chapter 1 about obtaining medical clearance (and having a stress test, if necessary). Select exercises and activities that you think you will enjoy. Begin your program cautiously. There is no need to try to make up overnight for the sedentary ways of a lifetime. By starting out too rigorously, you can incur an injury or suffer some discomfort that may discourage you from continuing to exercise. By beginning at very low levels of intensity and duration, you may successfully avoid injuries to muscles and joints that are unaccustomed to even moderate stress. Once your body has become used to low levels of activity, you can begin to increase your exercise by applying the principles of progressive overload outlined in Chapter 2.

What can be done to prevent or reduce the stiffness and pain in muscles and joints that often occur with advancing age? Pain and loss of flexibility in the joints are usually caused by the shortening and tightening of the connective tissue in the ligaments, tendons, muscles, and joints. This can occur at any age when the muscles and joints remain inactive for a significant amount of time. Flexibility exercises such as those in the stretching model program in Chapter 7 can help to reverse or reduce this process. So can calisthenics and weight training exercises, if they are performed through the full range of motion of the joints involved. The more active you are, the less likely you are to have pain or difficulty of this sort. Walk, reach, bend, squat, stoop, and stretch whenever possible to help keep muscles and joints limber.

Doesn't aerobic capacity inevitably decrease with age? Yes. The maximum amount of oxygen you can utilize during strenuous work does usually decrease with age. But by following a sound CRE program (see Chapter 7), you can delay the decline and even improve your CRE.

11

Programs for Special Needs

Health limitations—whether permanent or temporary—are not necessarily a deterrent to exercise. Since the end of World War II, there has been wheelchair competition in basketball, and there are marathon competitors confined to wheelchairs. Skiers know of one-legged practitioners of the sport, and some baseball fans may remember Pete Gray, the one-armed major league outfielder who played for the old St. Louis Browns. Many blind athletes participate in sports such as golf, cross-country and Alpine skiing, wrestling, track, swimming, tandem bicycling, and rowing.

If you have been avoiding exercise because of health problems, perhaps such examples could get you to reconsider the possibility. Some ways to exercise despite disabilities or health limitations are reviewed in this chapter. The suggestions made about programs for special needs are intended as guidelines, not as models to follow in every detail. For one thing, people with certain diseases—arthritis, asthma, and diabetes, for example—require more or less continuous medical supervision and should not change their activity level or life-style without seeking medical advice. This chapter should not be considered a substitute for that. It's important for people with special health needs to keep in touch with their physician at regular intervals. But with a physician's advice, it's possible to freely adjust and adapt any of the exercise ideas in this chapter to meet particular needs.

Arthritis

Arthritis means joint inflammation. Several types of arthritis with varying degrees of severity afflict millions of Americans. Of various medications for relief of inflammation, aspirin is the drug most commonly prescribed for rheumatoid arthritis, a disease of unknown origin. Moist heat also helps to reduce pain. To maintain and improve joint flexibility, stretching exercises should be done regularly. Resistance exercises with weights or with a partner providing the resistance will maintain strength in the muscles surrounding the affected joint. Isometric exercise is helpful for muscular strength if pain is present or flexibility is lacking. Swimming and exercising in warm water are excellent (see aqua exercises in the Glossary of Exercises). These steps do not stop the progress of the disease, and sometimes surgical joint replacement becomes necessary.

Osteoarthritis—the most common form of arthritis—is the type of joint inflammation that afflicts many older persons. Some readers of *Consumer Reports* wrote that they credited exercise with helping them overcome the aches and pains of osteoarthritis. You can use the Glossary of Exercises to design your own program. Excessive body weight can make arthritis worse, so if your condition allows, consider a program to develop cardiorespiratory endurance (CRE), which will be useful in weight control.

Asthma

People who have asthma are susceptible to attacks of shortness of breath, wheezing, and coughing. These attacks are frequently brought on by exposure to various allergens and sometimes may be psychosomatic in origin. But they are also often associated with exercise.

Recent studies indicate that a significant factor in exercise-induced asthma may be increased breathing in of cold air. Under normal conditions, the air we breathe reaches the passages of the respiratory tract only after passing rather slowly through the entire airway. Air enters the nose or mouth, continues through the trachea and bronchi, and finally fills the smallest branches of the bronchial tree—the bronchioles and air sacs. The inhaled air is thus warmed before it reaches the smaller airway passages. In exercise-induced asthma, smooth-muscle spasm in the bronchioles occurs as a result of the increased movement of cold air in the respiratory system.

Asthmatics can alter the conditions likely to trigger an attack by undertaking a program of cardiorespiratory conditioning to increase aerobic capacity. The better your aerobic capacity, the less likely you are to wheeze during exercise. In fact, several studies have substantiated a decrease in the number of attacks experienced by asthmatics during a swimming program.

In very cold weather, of course, even well-conditioned asthmatics may be unable to prevent an attack. Asthmatics can best cope with outdoor winter exertion by wrapping a scarf loosely around the nose and mouth or by wearing a ski mask, thus warming the air slightly before it is inhaled. It would be even better to confine exercise in winter to a warm moist atmosphere. Swimming in a heated indoor pool, for example, is ideal for asthmatics, especially in winter.

If you have asthma, note that acute attacks are more likely to occur if you exercise only occasionally. With regular exercise, you can slowly and gradually increase your CRE and build up your resistance to the attacks.

Here are some guidelines for a conditioning program for asthmatics, which emphasizes CRE training.

■ Start out slowly, if you're a beginner, until you learn your capabilities and limitations.

■ Begin with a five-to-ten minute warm-up, which should include cardiorespiratory activity (easy jogging or running in place); muscular endurance exercises (push-ups, pull-ups, sit-ups); and flexibility exercises (see stretching model program in Chapter 7).

■ End with a five-to-ten minute cool-down after each workout.

■ Good activities for asthmatics include interval training and games that are interrupted by periods of inactivity.

■ To get a training effect, cardiorespiratory activity periods should be thirty to forty-five minutes long, three times a week.

■ It helps to breathe with pursed lips (as if you were going to whistle). Breathing like this is easiest if you do it when standing up with the torso tilted slightly forward.

■ Wheezing episodes may occur fairly frequently during the first few weeks of training, but after the third week or so, wheezing generally diminishes.

■ Avoid outdoor activities during the pollen season, when there is air-borne mold, or if there is a sudden change to cold weather.

■ Avoid exercising in a dry or dusty indoor environment.

Children with asthma

Bronchial asthma is the most common chronic illness of childhood. This need not mean children have to be treated as invalids, however. But an effective exercise program for asthmatic children requires the cooperation of the physician, parent, child, and school. Every effort should be made to minimize restrictions for asthmatic children so they can take part in sports and physical education activities. Because the emotional aspects of competitive athletics may precipitate asthma attacks, body-contact sports should not be encouraged for children with severe asthma.

Cardiovascular problems

Exercise can play an important role in prevention and rehabilitation of some heart and circulatory ailments. But as must be obvious, physical activity is but one technique among many measures that may be helpful in dealing with these problems.

Angina pectoris

Angina pectoris (literally, chest pain), frequently referred to as "angina," may occur when a coronary artery fails to provide the amount of oxygen required by the heart muscles. As your physician will probably tell you, angina is a sign of coronary heart disease. After an angina attack, you may be asked to make some changes in your life-style, such as weight loss, less dietary fats, regular medication, giving up cigarettes, and participation in a regular exercise program to enhance CRE. The exercise will help you to increase your aerobic capacity, burn calories, and possibly feel better.

Heart attack

If you have had a heart attack, you can be certain that your physician will recommend that you make some changes in your life-style to try to reduce the risk of a second attack and to help you return to your previous (or higher) level of activity. Joseph S. Alpert, M.D., in *The Heart Attack Handbook,* states that, "These changes include stopping cigarette smoking, losing weight and decreasing physical and psychological stress. Other specific changes may include medication to regulate the heart, blood pressure or blood cholesterol level, and a graded exercise program."

After recovery from a heart attack, physicians generally recommend an organized exercise program such as those sponsored by hospitals, "Y" associations, community centers, colleges, and private cardiac rehabilitation facilities. These programs are carried out under medical supervision. The exercise facility should contain emergency medical equipment and all personnel should be thoroughly trained in cardiopulmonary resuscitation.

Your exercise prescription should be individually designed. The specific program should be devised by a qualified exercise physiologist in accordance with a physician's recommendations. A carefully monitored cardiac stress test provides the guidelines. Intensity should be based on a percentage of your maximum heart rate and your exercise benefit zone should be clearly defined. Your pulse may be monitored manually or by radio telemetry. Duration and frequency should follow the guidelines spelled out in Chapters 2 and 3. Activities should emphasize development of CRE but may include some work on muscular fitness, perhaps as part of the warm-up and cool-down. Isometric or heavy-resistance muscle work should be kept to a minimum.

If you are highly motivated, you may do well on a home program. After consultation with your physician, simply stick with the exercise regimen recommended to you. Contact your physician if you wish to change your activity or need recommendations about how to achieve progressive overload.

Also clear with your physician participation in sports and games. Your capacity for these activities will depend on the level of fitness you achieve through your conditioning program. If you reach high levels of conditioning without symptoms, your physician may permit you to engage in vigorous sports.

Hypertension

As many know only too well, hypertension (high blood pressure) is a common and potentially serious health problem. Although the causes of the disease remain unresolved, it can be controlled by diet, exercise, and medication. It would not be accurate to say that exercise alone can be used to treat hypertension.

One study of twenty-three hypertensive and twenty-two normotensive (normal blood pressure) men thirty-five to sixty-one years old showed that after six months of a CRE activity twice a week, the hypertensive group significantly reduced both resting systolic (upper figure) and diastolic (lower figure) blood pressure.

In another study of fifty-five hypertensive men, seventeen to fifty-nine years old who jogged for ten weeks, both resting systolic and diastolic blood pressure were reduced significantly. In another ten-week jogging study, however, no reduction in blood pressure resulted. On the question as to whether CRE training reduces blood pressure, authorities seem to agree that if one's blood pressure is generally normal to begin with, fitness training can do little to reduce it further.

Using medical records on blood pressure, researchers questioned 1,700 males sixteen years old and over regarding their level of physical activity. It was found that the more active men, regardless of age, had significantly lower systolic and diastolic blood pressure. Body fat correlated positively with blood pressure: The higher the body fat, the higher the blood pressure.

There is fairly good evidence to indicate that with *moderate* hypertension, regular exercise over a long period of time has a tendency to decrease blood pressure, although that is certainly not guaranteed. People on blood pressure medication who plan to begin an exercise regimen should be sure to check with their doctor: The medication may have to be reduced in order to offset the effect of the training program. Of the exercise regimens likely to be prescribed, CRE programs seem the most appropriate. Weight training, isometric exercise, and calisthenics may be risky; consult your physician before beginning such a program. An overall treatment program must be carried out under a physician's care, of course.

Diabetes

Diabetes mellitus is a chronic disorder of the metabolism of sugar, protein, and fat. It is due to a deficiency of insulin, a hormone made in the pancreas. If some combination of genetic, immune, and possibly viral factors make your pancreas unable to produce insulin, you have Type 1, or insulin-dependent, diabetes. (The disease was formerly known as juvenile-onset diabetes, even though it can appear at any age.) Type 1 diabetics must take one or more injections of insulin every day. If insulin is withheld for any reason, diabetic ketoacidosis, coma, and death may occur in a few days. If too much insulin is taken, the consequences can be equally dangerous: Severe hypoglycemia (low blood sugar) can produce convulsions and coma.

It is a well-accepted premise that better control of Type 1 diabetes may prevent such complications as eye, kidney, and nerve damage. The balance between insulin and diet is the key to achieving control of diabetes and preventing complications. Many Type 1 diabetics are now monitoring their own blood sugars several times a day, and, with the help of their physicians, regulating their insulin accordingly.

Type 1 diabetics usually find that the more they exercise the less insulin they require. Although the role of exercise in the balance between insulin and diet has long been recognized, the exact mechanism has only recently been explained. It now seems clear from studies in humans as well as in animals that exercising the muscles into which the insulin has been injected speeds its absorption into the bloodstream.

In some cases, absorption of insulin from strenuously exercised muscles can take place so rapidly that hypoglycemia can result. Moving the injection site away from the exercising muscle groups may eliminate this problem in some diabetics; in others, this approach may not be effective. Type 1 diabetics must therefore take a great many things into consideration when they begin an exercise program.

Only about 20 percent of diabetics can be classified as having Type 1. The rest have Type 2, or noninsulin-dependent, diabetes. Formerly known as maturity-onset or adult-onset diabetes, Type 2 is probably almost entirely genetic in origin. In these patients, the pancreas may produce normal or even above-normal amounts of insulin, yet blood sugar levels rise and the clinical condition known as diabetes follows, despite the seeming paradox of elevated blood levels of insulin. Type 2 diabetics lack sufficient insulin receptors on their body cells. These cell surface receptors facilitate entry of glucose into the cell where it can be used effectively.

The complications of Type 2 differ somewhat from those of Type 1, although considerable overlap is common. They include coronary heart disease, cerebrovascular disease (stroke), and peripheral vascular disease (gangrene). It is particularly important to regulate Type 2 diabetes and guard against the onset of complications.

Obviously, many Type 2 patients do not require insulin injections since they have an adequate supply of their own insulin. Recently some doctors have used oral hypoglycemic agents such as tolbutamide (Orinase) to lower the blood sugar levels, but use of these agents is controversial. However, there is a way to improve Type 2 diabetes that does not require any medicine. The beneficial effects of exercise are evident in the successful control of Type 2 diabetes. By exercising and also losing weight in the process, Type 2 diabetics—most of whom are obese—can increase the number of insulin receptors on their body cells, and thus facilitate the action of their own insulin. When this occurs, blood sugar returns toward normal and no oral medications are required.

If you have diabetes, you should consult your physician about suitable exercises. CRE should be the basis of your program, with activities chosen for their fitness benefits. But the ones selected should also be enjoyable for you so that you will get enough pleasure from the program to want to continue it.

A CRE program with an exercise benefit zone (EBZ, see pages 62–66) of 50 to 70 percent of the maximum heart rate can be beneficial. Even poorly conditioned diabetics may improve after brisk walking for thirty minutes, three times a week. With activities such as cross-country skiing, hiking, or long-distance running, it's important to observe proper precautions as well as adhere to the principles of gradual progressive overload. Learn how a particular exercise affects your body before you risk being out alone on a trail in winter or on a remote country road. Be sure you wear or carry a tag or card that identifies you as a diabetic in case of an emergency far from home and friends. Adequate nutrition is particularly important for diabetics on medication, so carry snacks with you that can raise your blood sugar quickly should the need arise. Candy and dried fruits are especially useful because of their high sugar content, small size, and light weight.

Orthopedic problems

There is a wide range of orthopedic problems—injuries and disabilities affecting the muscles, bones, and joints. Among the more common are muscle sprains and strains, fractured bones, torn cartilages, joint separations and dislocations, ruptured tendons, and tendinitis.

There is no substitute for competent medical care when such ailments occur. At some stage in your therapy, your doctor will probably prescribe reconditioning exercise. The exercise may substitute for surgery, follow the removal of a cast, or aim to recondition muscles and joints after surgery. A balanced program (to the extent permitted by the injury) is essential if you are to maintain and improve your fitness level. You may, of course, have to adapt your program considerably to protect the injured part. An injured wrist, for example, may mean you have to give up tennis. But you might be able to use a stationary bicycle or take up jogging. A leg injury may require exercise while seated or lying down. In any case, your program should include two aspects—general conditioning and a specific therapeutic exercise for the injured part.

Probably the most common orthopedic complaint is low-back pain. Millions of Americans have suffered at least one episode of severe, prolonged pain in the small of the back. And a good number are under medical treatment for chronic low-back pain. The causes of all this suffering vary, but most authorities agree that exercise can help solve many back problems. And a few simple changes in routine body mechanics may also help. If you are susceptible to backaches, try one or more of the following suggestions.

■ Avoid prolonged standing. If you must stand, support your weight mainly on your heels, with one or both knees slightly flexed.

■ Walk with your toes pointed ahead.

■ Avoid high-heeled shoes.

■ Always sit with your lower back slightly rounded and with your feet flat on the floor—especially during prolonged sitting, as during a plane ride or auto trip.

■ Avoid lying flat on your stomach or back. If you must lie on your back, place a pillow under your knees. Lying curled on one side is usually the most comfortable position for people with low-back problems.

■ To lift a load from the floor, squat with both knees bent and at least one foot flat on the floor. Keep your back straight. Always bend the knees: Never bend straight over from the waist. Never lift a load above your waist. Keep your hips and knees bent a little so that the weight of the load is not borne by the lower back.

Exercises for lower back

Four major muscle groups affect your back: the abdominal muscles, the muscles along the spine, the side muscles, and the muscles of the hips. The exercise program illustrated below will stretch and strengthen each of these muscle groups. Some people who suffer from low-back pain have also found aqua exercises to be helpful (see the Glossary of Exercises).

Before undertaking an exercise program for the lower back, it is important to check with your doctor. And once you start exercising, you should keep at it. Always perform the exercises slowly and progress very gradually until you are able to do ten repetitions of each exercise. This process may take two to three weeks.

---

1. Alternate knee-to-chest
(See Glossary 13E)

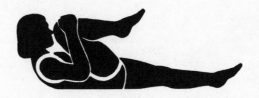

---

2. Leg cross-overs
(See Glossary 15E)

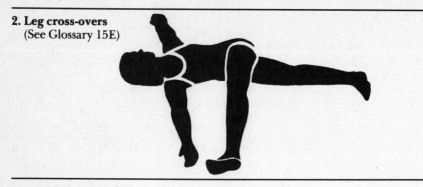

3. Double knee-to-chest
(See Glossary 14E)

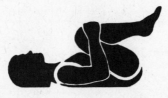

4. Sit-up
(See Glossary 24E)

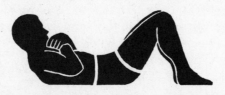

5. Back extension
(See Glossary 20E)

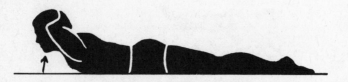

6. Alternate hip extension
(See Glossary 21E)

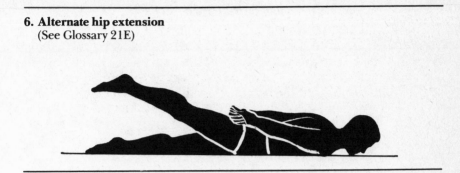

Postsurgical rehabilitation

Any active person confined to bed for even a short time is bound to suffer the effects of deconditioning. As a result of prolonged inactivity, all the fitness components deteriorate. And the longer the period of inactivity, the greater the degree of deconditioning. Because of this, even patients who have had major surgery are encouraged to begin some form of exercise almost as soon as they come out of anesthesia.

Recovery is hastened if the patient begins to exercise while still confined to bed. Various forms of flexing, stretching, toe wiggling, knee bending, and respiratory exercises such as deep breathing and coughing can help the patient avoid muscle atrophy as well as lessen the chance of blood clots and pneumonia. A graduated regimen of cardiorespiratory conditioning usually begins with legs dangling over the side of the bed. Then, with help, the patient is encouraged to take a few steps and to sit in a chair while the bed is made or while eating a meal. Soon the walking distance is increased, with or without the help, until the patient can pace up and down the hospital corridors, slowly building up muscular and cardiorespiratory endurance. Current practice demonstrates that the sooner activity is initiated, the shorter the period of convalescence will be.

If you are recuperating at home, discuss your exercise plans with your doctor to be sure your program is suited to your condition. When starting a postsurgical CRE program, limit your activity to keep your heart rate below the EBZ—50 to 70 percent of your maximum heart rate, perhaps. After your system has made the necessary adaptations, you may be ready to increase the intensity of your workout. Muscular exercise should also begin well below your presurgery fitness levels. Gradually increase the intensity, duration, and frequency, in accord with suggestions made in Chapters 2 and 3. During the early postsurgical stages, it is best to break up each day's workout into several short sessions. That way you don't risk becoming overtired or discouraged by doing too much at one time. Gradual progressive overload is especially important in the early stages of recuperation from illness or surgery.

Pregnancy

If you were exercising before your pregnancy, keep to your regular program, modifying it as your body tells you to. Always let your doctor know what your program consists of —the type of exercises, frequency, duration, etc. Or you may want to try the program below in place of your regular one. If you have not been exercising regularly before your pregnancy and you want to start, you must first get your doctor's approval.

The following program is especially designed for pregnant exercisers—both veteran exercisers and beginners.

■ Warm up for five to ten minutes by walking—slow to brisk—while swinging your arms.

■ Perform each of the twelve exercises (see below) daily, as described. Do them slowly and rhythmically. Avoid strain and stop before you feel fatigued. They should take from fifteen to twenty minutes.

■ Do the Kegel exercise (see below) to strengthen the pelvic floor.

■ Select a CRE program from those recommended in Chapter 3 or choose one of the CRE model programs in Chapter 7. Always use your EBZ as your guide. If you have been relatively sedentary, the walking model program would be an excellent choice.

Kegel exercise

The pelvic floor, which supports the pelvic organs including the bladder, uterus, and rectum, requires strengthening to prevent urinary leakage and uterine prolapse. The Kegel exercise, practiced during and after pregnancy, is excellent for strengthening the pelvic floor. This exercise may make delivery less uncomfortable because it increases the ability to relax the sphincter muscles. Prenatal training of the pelvic floor muscles will make it easier to retrain these muscles after delivery. Alternately tighten and relax the sphincter muscles of the perineal area—the muscles that surround the vaginal and urethral sphincter in front and the anal sphincter at the rear. (Stopping the urinary stream several times while urinating will give you a good idea of what happens when the sphincters are tightened.)

As a very private exercise, it can be done (even when not urinating) wherever you are, and only you will know it. Do about five in a series, holding each contraction for about five seconds. Do at least fifty a day.

Pregnancy exercises

The following series of twelve exercises takes about fifteen to twenty minutes to perform. You can do them daily, if you wish.

---

1. Groin stretch (helps make the delivery position more comfortable)
Start by holding your ankles with the soles of your feet touching each other. Lean forward and press your knees down with your elbows, feeling

a gentle stretch in your groin and inner thighs. Hold the position for ten to thirty seconds. Repeat three times.

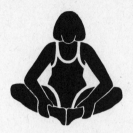

2. Single knee tuck (stretches lower back to help prevent or reduce back pain)

Start on your back with knees bent and the soles of your feet flat. Bring one knee to your chest, feeling a gentle stretch of the lower back. Relax the lower back as you hold for ten seconds. Switch knees and repeat the entire cycle three times.

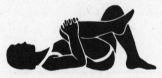

3. Double knee tuck (stretches lower back to help reduce low-back pain)

See illustration for single knee tuck, above. Start on your back with knees bent and soles flat. Grip both knees and bring your knees to your chest. Keep the back relaxed as you hold the gentle stretch for three to ten seconds. Repeat three times.

4. Pelvic tilting on back (to strengthen the abdominal muscles)

Start on your back with knees bent. Place one hand in the hollow of your back, the other on the rim of the hip. Slowly tighten the abdominal and buttock muscles by pushing down on your hand with the small of your back. Rock the baby back into the pelvic cradle as you roll your hips back gently. Breathe out as you contract the abdominal muscles. Hold the

237

contraction for three to six seconds then relax as you breathe in. Keep your back flat throughout. Repeat three to five times.

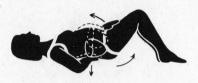

5. Hamstring stretch (to stretch the hamstring muscles)

Start with one leg straight, the other tucked in. Reach for the ankle of the extended leg, feeling the gentle stretch of the muscles in the back of the thigh. Hold the stretch for ten to thirty seconds. Switch legs and repeat the entire cycle three times.

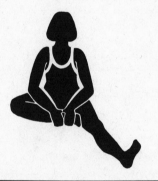

6. Sit-back (for abdominal strength and endurance)

Start in an upright sitting position. Reach forward with your arms and sit back to a 45° angle. Hold the V-like position for three to six seconds. Repeat three times.

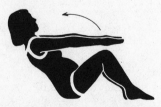

7. Chest push (for strength and endurance of the chest muscles)

Start with your elbows bent and palms together. Press your palms firmly together so that you can feel the tightening of the pectoral muscles under the breasts. Hold the press for three to six seconds. Repeat three times.

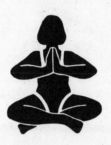

8. Pelvic tilting on all fours (to strengthen abdominal muscles)

Start in a kneeling position with your arms extended for support. Pull your back and pelvis up into a catlike position. Hold for three to six seconds and relax to the starting position, but never let your spine sag. Repeat three times.

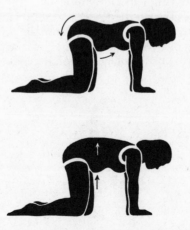

9. Modified sit-up (to strengthen abdominal muscles)

Start flat on your back with knees bent. Tilt your pelvis up, flattening your back. Extend your arms and slowly curl up. Tuck your chin in and come up one vertebra at a time, as you lift your head first and then your shoulders. Stop when you can see your heels and hold for three to six seconds before returning to the starting position. Repeat three times.

Don't do this exercise if your abdominal muscles have separated (come to a point).

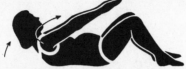

10. Back arch (to strengthen lower-back muscles)

Start on your back with knees bent and arms flat alongside. Do a pelvic tilt and then lift your tailbone, buttocks, and lower back from the floor. Hold this position for three to six seconds, with your weight resting on your feet, arms, and shoulders. Return to starting position and repeat three times.

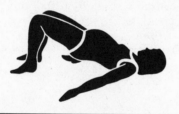

11. Squat (to strengthen thigh and hip muscles)

Start with your feet flat on the floor, squatting half-way down. Hold for three to six seconds, then stand up. Eventually go into full squat. If necessary, have a partner hold your hands to assist with balance. Repeat three times. (If you have knee problems, limit movement to half squat.)

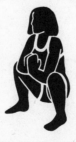

12. Wall push-away (for strength and endurance of the arms and shoulders and for flexibility of the Achilles tendon)

Start supporting yourself with your arms extended against the wall. Bend your arms, allowing your head and upper body to slowly come toward the wall. Hold this position for ten seconds so that you can feel the stretch of your calves and Achilles tendon. Push away slowly to starting position. Repeat three times.

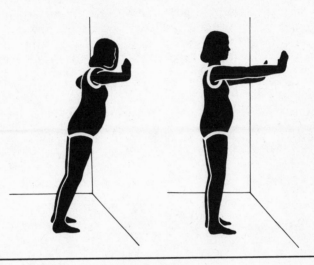

Depression

Depression is one of the most common emotional problems in the United States.It has been reported that up to 10 percent of the population, if tested on a standard depression questionnaire, would score in the "depressed" range. Levels of depression vary from the mild blues to suicidal attitudes. Many depressions are self-limiting—they usually come to an end on their own sooner or later. Methods of treatment vary and may include antidepressant drugs, psychotherapy, and electroshock therapy.

Various attempts to study the effects of physical activities on moderate depression have produced unclear results. Some investigators have concluded that such activities as jogging, wrestling, and tennis have been effective in some cases but not in others. Some psychotherapists reportedly use exercise as part of their treatment of patients with depression. And there are any number of subjective reports of psychological benefits.

Definitive answers about the effect of exercise on depression must await additional scientific evidence. Questions yet to be answered revolve around whether the reported benefits can be substantiated, and whether they are due to physiological changes, increased self-esteem because of improvement in fitness, being part of a group, or some factor intrinsic to the activity itself. But if exercise makes you feel better, then by all means exercise. There is no indication that pleasurable physical activity will cause emotional problems—and it may even help you.

Associations for the handicapped

The list below includes organizations for handicapped people who are interested in sports and other athletic activities. The names of many of these organizations are self-explanatory. For others, a brief explanation appears in parentheses following the entry for the organization. Addresses are included so you can write for information. (This list was compiled from the *Encyclopedia of Associations*, 17th edition, 1983.)

American Athletic Association for the
   Deaf
10604 East 95th Street Terrace
Kansas City, Missouri 64134

American Blind Bowling Association
150 North Bellaire Avenue
Louisville, Kentucky 40206

American Blind Skiing Foundation
610 South William Street
Mount Prospect, Illinois 60056

American Wheelchair Bowling
   Association
6718 Pinehurst Drive
Evansville, Indiana 47711

Blind Outdoor Leisure Development
533 East Main Street
Aspen, Colorado 81611

Handicapped Boaters Association
P.O. Box 1134
Ansonia Station
New York, New York, 10023

Healthsports, Inc.
1455 West Lake Street
Minneapolis, Minnesota 55408
(for visually and physically disabled
   interested in cross-country skiing
   and other sports)

International Committee of Sports
   for the Deaf
Gallaudet College
Washington, D.C. 20002

National Association for Disabled
   Athletes
2069 Fletcher Avenue
Fort Lee, New Jersey 07024

National Association of Sports
   for Cerebral Palsied
c/o Craig A. Huber
66 East 34th Street
New York, New York 10016

National Deaf Bowling
   Association
9244 East Mansfield Avenue
Denver, Colorado 80237

National Foundation for Happy
   Horsemanship for
   the Handicapped
Box 462
Malvern, Pennsylvania 19355

National Foundation of
   Wheelchair Tennis
3857 Birch Street
Newport, California 92660

National Handicapped Sports and
Recreation Association
P.O. Box 18664
Capitol Hill Station
Denver, Colorado 80218

National Wheelchair Athletic
Association
2107 Templeton Gap Road
Suite C
Colorado Springs, Colorado 80907

National Wheelchair Basketball
Association
110 Seaton Building
University of Kentucky
Lexington, Kentucky 40506

National Wheelchair Softball
Association
P.O.Box 737
Sioux Falls, South Dakota 57101

North American Riding for the
Handicapped Association
P.O. Box 100
Ashburn, Virginia 22011

One-Arm Dove Hunt Association
Box 582
Olney, Texas 76374
(for amputees interested in shooting
competitions, dove hunting)

Special Olympics
1701 K Street, N.W.
Suite 203
Washington, D.C. 20006
(for the retarded)

U.S. Association for Blind Athletes
55 West California Avenue
Beach Haven, New Jersey 08008

United States Deaf Skiers Association
159 Davis Avenue
Hackensack, New Jersey 07601

Wheelchair Motorcycle Association
101 Torrey Street
Brockton, Massachusetts 02401

12

Training Tips

When you do exercises on your own—jogging, swimming, or weight training, say—there are bound to be times when you wish you had a coach, a trainer, or a physician to advise you. You may only want reassurance, or perhaps an evaluation of your progress. Some of your questions on specific aspects of training may have been answered already in earlier chapters. In this chapter are answers to questions that came from readers of *Consumer Reports* as well as a sampling of the kinds of questions our senior authors have been asked repeatedly over the years.

Is it safe to exercise outdoors in the cold? With good judgment and the right clothing, most people can safely—and enjoyably—exercise even in subfreezing temperatures. People with heart conditions, however, should not do strenuous exercise outdoors in very cold weather without discussing it first with their physician. The average person will find that the body's heating system, like its cooling system, is very effective. When you run, you burn calories. This raises the temperature of the blood circulating through the body and thus warms the body. The hardest thing about exercising in cold weather is getting up the courage to go out the door. If you dress to keep heat from escaping, you may be surprised how warm you'll be even on the coldest days.

Is there any harm in breathing freezing air into the lungs—especially through the mouth? No, unless you're asthmatic (see page 227). By the time the cold air gets to your lungs, it has had ample time to be warmed. Cold dry air may feel irritating to the throat, however, but you can avoid that by wearing a ski mask, wrapping a scarf around your face, or wearing a hooded sweat shirt and tightening the drawstrings so that the hood covers most of your face.

How can frostbite be prevented? Frostbite is a condition in which body tissues are damaged or destroyed by freezing. The length of time you are exposed, the wind chill factor, and how much moisture there is in the air and on the skin all affect your chances of getting frostbite. The most important element in prevention is proper clothing. The nose, ears, fingers, toes, cheeks, and penis are most vulnerable and should be carefully protected. The first sign of impending frostbite is a blotch of snow-white skin (usually on the nose or cheek). Covering the spot with a gloved hand for a short time will usually restore the circulation and color—no need for alarm at this point. Not to be ignored are later warning symptoms of numbness, tingling, and pain accompanied by a red, flushed appearance of the skin. Burning or itching may develop, and eventually the area becomes totally insensitive.

At this point, it's important to warm the injured tissue rapidly and gently by applying warm water (about 105°F). *Don't rub the skin with snow!* This folk remedy can be dangerous. Protect the injured area from further cold, and see a physician as soon as possible.

What should be worn when exercising in cold weather? It depends on air temperature, wind speed, humidity, and the intensity of your exercise. An air temperature of 40°F on a calm day is one thing, but if there is an accompanying wind speed of 15 miles per hour, the effective temperature would be 22°F. So you must dress taking into account the wind chill factor as well as the temperature. The intensity of your exercise is also important. The harder you work, the more calories you burn and the more heat your body produces. Activities such as running, bicycling, and cross-country skiing continuously burn a lot of calories. If you overdress for such activities, you will sweat excessively and the chilling effect of your own perspiration may cause serious problems.

The trick is, of course, to dress in layers. The first layer should be nonirritating, and, if possible, made of cotton. A new alternative is polypropylene, which is believed to draw moisture away from the skin. Over tee shirt and running shorts can go a layer of wool, which is a good insulator even when wet. Top it off with a tightly woven cotton windbreaker or a nylon one of a type that allows perspiration to filter to the outside. Hats and mittens (or gloves) are essential to prevent the loss of body heat. You can add or subtract many kinds of clothing depending on the weather. On long-distance outings (cross-country skiing, for example), you may need a small backpack to carry the extra layers as your body warms up and you begin to strip down, or to carry warm clothing to put on when you stop to rest or in case of injury. (See also page 251.)

Is it all right to run in rain or snow? Fine, if you enjoy it. But keep a few precautions in mind. With most waterproof clothing, your body heat cannot easily escape and your perspiration cannot evaporate. Soon you may find sweat trickling down inside your clothes. Choose rainwear that "breathes," such as clothing made of Gore-Tex, a waterproofing product, or that has sufficient ventilation to allow air to circulate around your body and get through to the atmosphere. In snow or light rain, a water-repellent nylon sweat or warm-up suit will probably keep you dry enough. Be alert for icy patches and be prepared for the possibility of reduced traction. Obviously you should cut down on your usual speed when running in wet weather.

Is it true you burn more calories in cold weather than in moderate or warm weather? Yes. Your body has to work harder to keep warm, and so more calories are used.

Can you acclimate yourself to exercising in the cold? Apparently there is some evidence that people who exercise outdoors in winter adapt to the cold. One study indicated that after fourteen to sixteen hours of daily exposure for about two weeks, the study subjects felt considerably more comfortable in the cold, had warmer hands and feet, and shivered less than they did before.

How does hot weather and high humidity affect exercisers? In brief periods of strenuous activity, exercisers are little affected by extremes in temperature and humidity. But in prolonged vigorous exercise (such as jogging), they can be severely impaired. During hot weather, the circulatory system must divert significant quantities of blood to the skin, where heat is released in the form of sweat. As sweat evaporates, it cools both the skin and the blood circulating near the body surface. This cooled blood then continues to circulate, lowering the body temperature. Exercise makes a conflicting demand upon the circulation. During activity to improve cardiorespiratory endurance, the circulatory system must deliver large quantities of oxygen to the muscles and continue to do so as long as the activity persists. These competing responsibilities of the circulatory system are further complicated by extremely high temperature and humidity. The hotter the weather, the more water the body loses in the form of sweat. And the more humid the weather, the less efficient the sweating mechanism is in lowering the body temperature, since evaporation takes place less rapidly when the air is already loaded with moisture. The combination of increased cardiorespiratory activity and loss of body fluid presents a number of health hazards to persons who exercise strenuously in hot humid weather.

How can one recognize and treat the different forms of heat disorders? A person with mild *heat fatigue* feels extremely tired, has a rapid heart rate, and performs physical and mental tasks poorly. You can easily treat heat fatigue by having the person stop exercising and rest in a shady cool location, preferably one with a breeze.

Without treatment, heat fatigue may progress to *heat exhaustion,* during which the body temperature rises, blood pressure drops, pulse becomes rapid and weak, and sweating increases, which causes the skin to become cold and clammy. Persons with heat exhaustion look pale, may complain of headache, be mentally confused, vomit, or even lose consciousness. They should be made to lie down in a cool shady place and, if conscious and alert, drink plenty of fluids to replace the water lost by excessive sweating. It also helps to apply cool wet compresses and to fan them.

Heat cramps may result from loss of water and salt after prolonged exercise in hot weather. This too is easily remedied with rest and replacement of fluids.

The most extreme result of heat exposure is *heat stroke,* a medical emergency that requries the immediate attention of a physician. Heat stroke is a condition in which sweating is diminished or altogether absent, body temperature goes dangerously high, the skin appears hot, dry, and flushed, and respirations are deep and rapid. A person with heat stroke may be irritable or delirious, may suffer convulsions, lose consciousness, and even die. Until the doctor arrives, make every effort to lower body temperature by using ice cubes, immersion in a tub of cold water, using a fan, or cold wet compresses. Discontinue first aid as soon as the victim is awake and alert, but resume if body temperature rises again.

What is the best way to get used to exercising in hot weather? Take four to ten days to adjust to higher temperatures. Reduce your workouts by 50 percent, and give yourself a chance to cool off at intervals, if necessary. Gradually build up to your previous intensity and duration. It is no indication of weakness to cut down your activity level at the beginning of a heat spell or after a sudden move to a hot climate: It takes time for your body to adjust. When you become acclimated to hot humid weather, you will not only sweat sooner and more profusely than you did before your body adjusted, but you will produce sweat with a lower concentration of salt. With your body temperature being regulated more efficiently, your heart rate will slow down to previously normal levels.

Is it harder for women to exercise in hot weather than it is for men? No, despite some claims to the contrary. Men do seem to sweat more easily than women—that is, most men will begin to perspire before most women when performing a certain amount of exercise in an environment of a certain heat and humidity. This has led some authorities to conclude that men adapt to heat better than women. But other observers note that women can continue to work at a given intensity for a longer time in a given environment, and they conclude that women tolerate heat better than men. Conditioning can improve heat tolerance in both men and women. The more you work in warm environments, the more you become acclimated and the better your cooling system functions. Some people react to heat better than others, but there does not seem to be a consistent difference between men and women in this regard.

Isn't it harmful to drink water when exercising? No. Water not only helps your performance, it also helps prevent serious heat disorders. During prolonged exercise in hot weather, you may sweat anywhere from one to three quarts of water per hour. You must replace that fluid if you are to continue sweating and keep your body temperature within normal limits. Dehydration may set in after as little as thirty minutes of vigorous activity, especially if you have spent a long time warming up beforehand. The American College of Sports Medicine recommends that water stations be placed at two- or two-and-one-half-mile intervals along a race course of ten miles or more. Another recommendation is that runners should have something to drink at ten- or fifteen-minute intervals throughout a long-distance run. In any case, you should certainly have something to drink after an hour of strenuous activity.

It's a good idea to drink a glass or two of fluid ten or fifteen minutes *before* beginning exercise. But be careful not to drink too much, too soon before starting or a full bladder may make you uncomfortable.

At the end of a workout, you may find that you have lost a few pounds. This is entirely due to fluid loss, and is usually gained back after exercise.

Isn't it harmful to drink cold liquids when overheated from exercising? No. Studies do not support the widespread notion that drinking cold water causes stomach cramps or upsets the normal activity of the heart. Quite the contrary. There is evidence that cold fluids (45°F to 55°F) directly reduce internal body heat.

What are the rules for exercising in hot weather? The following hot weather exercise guidelines may be helpful.

■ Exercise in the early morning or late afternoon or evening, when ambient temperatures are lowest.

■ Drink a glass or two of fluid ten or fifteen minutes before exercising. How much you drink should depend on the duration and intensity of your planned activity as well as on the availability of fluid during the activity.

■ Avoid highly vigorous or competitive exercise in very warm weather—above 85°F, say, especially in humid weather.

■ Slow down or stop any activity if you begin to feel uncomfortable. Symptoms such as dry mouth, hot head, dizziness, disorientation, or muscle weakness may indicate the onset of a heat disorder.

■ Drink about one-half cup of fluid every ten or fifteen minutes during an activity that lasts more than fifty or sixty minutes—and even more frequently during high-intensity activity. Drink plain cold water, or fruit juice if you prefer.

■ Avoid taking salt pills or heavily salted food or drink before or during prolonged exercise. The body has its own defenses against excessive salt loss through sweating.

■ Keep a record of your early morning body weight (after rising and urinating but before breakfast) to determine whether weight lost through sweating has been restored. Weight loss of no more than about 3 percent (or 4 to 5 pounds for a 150-pound individual) is normal, and most of this weight is restored within twenty-four hours after activity. Excessive weight loss or weight loss that lasts for extended periods of time may indicate a need to reduce or discontinue activity temporarily.

■ Wear clothing that lets air circulate around the body. Avoid rubber suits (see page 80), which prevent the rapid evaporation of sweat.

Is there any advantage to drinking fluids containing "mineral-replacements" before, during, or after exercise? No. Manufacturers claim that these drinks assist athletic performance by replacing important mineral substances lost when you sweat. There is some evidence that preparations containing the same balance of salts found in sweat plus the large quantities of sugar found in commercial drinks may actually retard the emptying of the stomach and deprive the blood of needed water. If you insist on using one of the commercial drinks, at least dilute it with water—especially during vigorous prolonged exercise in hot weather.

Is it wise to exercise when you feel sick? It depends on whether you have a fever. Many authorities think exercising helps you feel better when you have a minor ailment, but most advise you to take it easy if you have a fever. If you do decide to exercise, it might be wise to reduce the intensity and duration of your workout. George Sheehan, M.D., a noted runner, advises that your resting pulse should be your guide if you are not sure you are well enough to exercise. If your heart rate is ten or more beats above your normal rate, you'd better omit your exercise session.

What precautions are necessary for exercising at high altitudes? Exercising at altitudes up to about 6,500 feet gives most people little or no trouble at all. At altitudes higher than that, the oxygen content of the air eventually decreases to the point that the working muscles become deprived of the oxygen they need. In other words, the cardiorespiratory system must work harder at higher altitudes than at sea level. At above 8,000 feet, some people experience difficulty even without exercise. They have trouble sleeping or getting up in the morning, and they may feel light-headed and nauseous. But as usual, the body adapts to changes in the environment. The symptoms of altitude illness generally disappear within two to five days. It takes time for acclimatization. If possible, ascend gradually, at a rate of one to three days for every 2,000 or 3,000 feet. Delay vigorous exercise until you are used to the altitude, and then begin at lower than usual intensity and duration, increasing gradually as you would when returning to an exercise program or beginning a new one. If you return to lower altitudes after an extended stay in the mountains you may find that the training effect you have achieved at high altitudes makes it easier for you to work at the same intensity at lower altitudes.

What about foot placement in jogging and running? For joggers and for runners at moderate speed, how the foot hits the ground can affect endurance and comfort. There is no question that a flat-footed strike or letting the heel hit first proves less tiring over a long distance than landing on the ball of the foot, as sprinters do. Runners who persist in routinely landing on the ball of the foot risk soreness from forcing the muscles to remain contracted over a long period of time.

Where are the best places to jog or run? Joggers and runners are not as free as walkers in selecting a setting for exercise. Walkers, because the activity requires less intensity, can usually get their exercise almost anywhere they choose. The simplest solution for a beginning runner faced with the problem of where to run is often the local high school outdoor track. Typically 440 yards, the track provides the beginner with a known distance so that performance can be measured and progress monitored. Some, however, may find that convenience and a smooth surface are not a sufficient counterbalance to the monotony of the track. Those who prefer a more varied setting risk twisted feet and ankles from irregular surfaces if they run on country roads or the sidewalks of a city. Pavement, even if smooth, can be jarring to a runner over time. Indoor tracks that are banked provide a special hazard: Running on a concave surface will exert uneven force on each foot. If you reverse your direction every now and then, you may be able to avoid discomfort and possible injury. Do not choose a hilly area if you are a beginning runner.

What is the best type of clothing to wear while walking, jogging, or running outdoors? Walkers can usually manage very nicely with any shoes that have adequate support. If readily available, hiking boots or shoes with thick soles and heels that provide good traction are ideal for walking. Regular walkers may want to consider investing in a pair of good quality training shoes used by joggers. Properly fitted, such shoes can make walking more pleasurable. Overdressing is a common mistake of the beginning walker. Avoid undue sweating by keeping clothes loose fitting and appropriate to the weather.

For joggers and runners, the proper footwear and clothing require careful consideration. In the very early stages of a jogging or running program, ordinary tennis shoes may suffice. To stick with sneakers over time, however, could lead to foot problems caused by inadequate support.

Even for the beginner, it pays to buy a pair of training shoes that fit well. But limit your selection to training shoes: The more delicate and light racing shoes are not for everyday use. Look for a lightweight shoe that's flexible, one that bends easily at the ball of the foot but is fairly rigid from the front of the arch to the heel. The shoe should provide cushioning that gradually thickens at the heel—to about twice the thickness of the front part of the shoe. That way the shoe will ease the stress on the heel as it strikes the ground. A firm heel counter helps keep the foot stable. The toe box should be comfortable, allowing for movement of the toes. Uppers should be soft. The best test of a shoe, no matter the price or its reputation, is how it fits you and how it works for you as a runner.

Not all runners use socks, but those who do usually prefer cotton or wool socks. Nylon tends to retain heat and moisture, increasing the possibility of blisters. Calf-length tubes provide more protection in winter than ankle socks. For some runners, two pairs of socks help prevent blisters: first a lightweight cotton pair and then a thicker pair. Others find that two pairs of socks cramp the foot. A new alternative is socks made of polypropylene, which is supposed to let the perspiration escape and so keep your feet dry.

On a cool day, a sweat suit can be handy. The old gray model is just as functional as the sleek new warm-up suits—and a lot less costly. During the winter months, mittens will help retain body heat more than gloves. Some people, especially those tending to baldness, like to use a cap year-round. In winter, a cap provides warmth and in summer, protection from the heat of the sun. Ski caps in extremely cold weather are useful because they can double as face masks.

Cotton shorts and shirts absorb sweat more efficiently than nylon clothing, but nylon can be laundered more easily. You can even take nylon shorts and a shirt into the shower and wash off the sweat as you soap up.

If you run after dark, wear reflectors so as to be visible to motorists.

What about jogging in a smoggy city? Air pollution in cities like Los Angeles may make exercising uncomfortable and even dangerous at times. And some people question whether the risks of running where there is a high concentration of automobile traffic outweigh the benefits of the exercise itself. Of course, no one should exercise outdoors during a smog alert or when air quality is downright poor. People with asthma, angina, emphysema, or other cardiorespiratory difficulties should avoid outdoor exertion when the air quality is only fair or poor. At any time, you should let your body help you decide how hard and how long your workout should be, or whether you should be out there running or playing at all. Any sign of eye irritation or respiratory discomfort may indicate that the air quality is poor and that you would be better off indoors jumping rope or pedaling a stationary bike. If you must exercise

251

outdoors in the smog, try to do it in the early morning or late evening, when lighter traffic, cooler temperatures, and lower humidity make the air quality better. Look for places to exercise away from heavy traffic, such as in parks, along river banks, or on residential streets rather than commercial or industrial thoroughfares. And if you must exercise alongside traffic, remember that pollution is lower where traffic keeps moving fast than where stop-and-go conditions increase the exhaust fumes.

Is taking protein, vitamin, and mineral supplements necessary for exercising? No. Unless you have specific symptoms of nutritional deficiency or unless you are certain that your dietary intake is inadequate, there should be no need for you to take any supplements at all. A balanced diet, one that provides a variety of foods from the four basic food groups, should be sufficient to meet your nutritional needs. If you wish to maintain your weight, however, you may have to increase your caloric intake, now that you are exercising regularly. Three foods each day from the meat group and three from the milk group should provide ample protein, even for a growing child. So pass up commercial protein supplements: They are unnecessary and costly.

The same advice holds for vitamins and minerals. There is no indication that exercise depletes a body's vitamin reserves. A varied selection from all the food groups provides sufficient vitamins for any normal person's needs. Although potassium and iron may, in some cases, be depleted by prolonged vigorous exercise, even they need not be replaced by using expensive commercial supplements. You can easily prevent the muscular weakness and fatigue associated with potassium or iron depletion. Just include plenty of vegetables, citrus fruits, and bananas in your daily diet to provide potassium, and include meat (particularly liver), fish, beans, green leafy vegetables, and dried fruits for iron.

Do protein, vitamin, and mineral supplements improve an athlete's performance? No. Athletes are always searching for a magic substance that will enhance their powers, and industry is always ready to profit from their quest. Despite the fact that there is no scientific evidence that the use of food supplements can improve athletic performance, many athletes—amateurs and professionals alike—are convinced that it can, and many "miraculous" formulations are on the market. The fact is that excessive amounts of niacin and vitamins A and D can be dangerous. The best nutritional aid to good health and athletic performance is a balanced diet.

Does caffeine help ward off exhaustion in prolonged endurance activity? The caffeine in two cups of coffee, taken sixty minutes before exercising, may delay the onset of exhaustion during extended activity, but there are risks to weigh against this supposed benefit. Caffeine acts as a stimulant on the brain and by so doing may forestall the sensation of fatigue. It stimulates cardiac output and muscular activity in general, and thus may help your body work harder for a time. But it also stimulates the production of urine—causing discomfort and inconvenience during a long-distance run, say.

What exactly is "carbohydrate loading"? Carbohydrate loading is a complicated technique sometimes used by long-distance runners to provide maximum energy during competition. You begin about seven days or so before your event by exercising for a sixty-to-ninety-minute (or more) workout—almost to the point of exhaustion. This depletes your muscle glycogen stores. For the next three or four days, you continue your regular training while severely limiting your carbohydrate intake (the source of glycogen). About three to four days before the competition, drastically increase your intake of carbohydrate—eating spaghetti, bread, potatoes, and the like. This results in high levels of muscle glycogen to sustain you through the latter part of the race, when fatigue usually sets in. In theory, and in carefully managed practice, carbohydrate loading leaves an athlete with very high levels of glycogen in the muscles, which can be called upon to meet the extreme demands of *prolonged* endurance competition. For anything but marathon competition, evidence is lacking that carbohydrate loading is beneficial.

What is the best time to eat before an athletic event and what should the meal consist of? If you eat a meal about three hours before an athletic event, you allow enough time for the food to be digested and absorbed, but not enough time for you to feel hungry again. Many athletes still prefer a hearty steak-and-potatoes kind of meal, but most authorities now advise a menu designed to avoid discomfort and improve performance. Foods likely to cause discomfort include anything that is hard to digest, such as foods rich in fat. Avoid foods such as cabbage, beans, and cauliflower, which cause gas to build up in the intestine. Stay away from foods you are not used to eating. Avoid foods high in protein and cellulose—such as meat and leafy vegetables—which may increase your need to urinate or defecate during your activity period. Spicy or salty food may make you thirsty and so should also be omitted.

Choose foods high in carbohydrate—spaghetti, bread, and potatoes—to give you quick energy without undue stress on the digestive system. Drink at least two or three glasses of fluid to be sure of adequate hydration. Table sugar or candy, though pure carbohydrate and regarded by many as a good source of instant energy, is of no proven value and may be detrimental. Excessive sugar may cause water retention in the digestive tract and thus interfere with the circulatory and heat regulatory systems so important in endurance exercise, especially in hot weather.

Is it wise to keep your weight down so you can compete in sports that are

based on weight classifications? No. For example, if muscular adolescents starve themselves to keep their weight down, their bodies are forced to obtain energy from muscle breakdown. The health risks connected with starvation or drying out in order to make the right weight classification (for a wrestling team, for instance) can be serious.

Do alcohol and exercise mix? Not very well. A small amount of alcohol— a glass of wine or beer at mealtime about three hours prior to exercise, say—is unlikely to have an adverse effect on activity. Larger amounts, however, can impair coordination or interfere with your exercise performance.

Alcohol is a central nervous system depressant that slows down the action of brain centers and reflex systems. The more you drink, the stronger the effects, although the effect of a given amount of alcohol may vary with such factors as the individual's body size, prior use of alcohol, and how fast you down a drink. One or two drinks may slightly reduce motor efficiency, while three or four drinks can result in significant loss of coordination. It takes about one hour, on average, to metabolize one ounce of alcohol.

Contrary to folklore, drinking alcohol before exercising in cold weather will not really warm you up. When you take a drink, the blood circulation to your extremities increases. This may make your hands and feet feel warm at first, but it ultimately has a chilling effect, since the heat is easily lost from the extremities. The anesthetic effect of alcohol may also dull the skin's sensitivity to cold and thus deprive you of an important warning signal of overexposure to the cold. Lastly, the loss of judgment and locomotor control possible with heavy alcohol use poses significant dangers for people who engage in high-risk activities such as water sports, mountain climbing, skiing, and biking.

Does smoking affect exercise? Cigarette smoking does indeed affect exercise. First, smoking constricts the bronchial tubes, the pathways through which oxygen and other gases enter and leave the body. This narrowing limits not only the amount of air your lungs can take in, but also the amount of carbon dioxide and other gases they can expel. Second, cigarette smoke contains carbon monoxide, a gas that can combine with the hemoglobin in red blood cells and take up space normally reserved for oxygen. The less oxygen your muscles get, the harder your cardiorespiratory system must work to try to supply it. Thus the more you smoke, the faster your heart beats. If you are a smoker, you can test this effect by taking your pulse both before and after you smoke a cigarette. You will probably note an increase of twelve to twenty beats per minute.

The immediate effects of smoking are only part of the problem. The lungs of chronic smokers lose some of the ability to process oxygen efficiently. Even without overt disease, smokers, on average, score lower in endurance performance than nonsmokers as a group. And after training, smokers do not improve as much as nonsmokers.

Can exercise help a smoker kick the habit? Many people—including many former smokers—think it can. The withdrawal symptoms you may experience when you give up smoking are, in many respects, the opposite of what exercisers often experience on a fitness program. Giving up a heavy tobacco habit may make you nervous, anxious, lethargic, and prone to headaches. Exercisers, however, often say they feel more relaxed, confident, and energetic, and that they have fewer headaches. In this view, therefore, the good effects of exercise may provide some sort of symptomatic protection against the bad effects of nicotine withdrawal. There is no evidence, however, that physical training has any direct physiological effect on tobacco dependence. Certainly, many people feel that the investment they make in an exercise program can act as additional motivation to reinforce their effort to stop smoking.

What causes a stitch in the side, and what can be done about it? The stitch in the side, the bane of many an athlete's existence, is a sharp pain at the bottom or side of the rib cage, usually on the right side. There are many possible explanations, but no one is absolutely sure what causes it. Some people think it results from spasms of the diaphragm. Others think side stitches are spasms of the abdominal muscles. One way to deal with this type of side stitch is to slow down or even stop exercising and push your fingertips into the pain site, while bending forward and exhaling. When the stitch occurs, breathe so that you thrust your abdomen out as you inhale. In general, try to strengthen your diaphragm and abdominal muscles by increasing your cardiorespiratory activity and also by doing bent-knee sit-ups. You might also try lying on your back with your legs raised, supporting your hips with your hands and keeping your legs moving ("riding a bicycle").

Some stitches seem to come from eating just before exercise. The theory goes that the blood supply is diverted from the intestinal tract to the exercising muscles, thus causing intestinal cramps. The obvious solution for this is to avoid eating for three hours prior to exercising. Still another theory is that gas in the lower intestinal tract causes stitches.

As usual when there are many "cures" for a problem, there is no one reliable solution. Take your pick and use whatever works best for you.

What can be done about blisters? A blister is a small pocket of fluid that accumulates just under the surface of the skin as a result of heat, friction, or irritation. Blisters frequently appear on the feet, particularly if shoes are too loose or if socks get wet. Prevent foot blisters by wearing clean, dry, well-fitting socks, and shoes that fit securely over the socks. The best way to treat blisters is to puncture them and let the fluid drain out. (Be sure your hands and the area around the blister are thoroughly clean.) Sterilize a needle by holding it in a flame until it turns red. Puncture the blister at several points around the edge and allow the fluid to drain; if necessary, press on the blister with a bit of sterile gauze to force the fluid out. Do not remove the skin from the blister. Cover the blister with a dry, sterile dressing of "nonstickable" gauze. Keep it clean, and change the dressing as necessary. Often it is possible to resume exercising immediately, as long as the bandage is tight and secure enough to stay in place and protect the wound. Consult a physician at the first sign of infection.

To prevent blisters, be sure to wear the right sort of shoes for your exercise, and be sure they fit correctly. Apply petroleum jelly to any irritated area as soon as you notice it. Avoid long periods of exercise with new shoes. Take time to break in a new pair. Try a ready-made blister-proof insole. Avoid exercising in wet shoes and socks. If you are a golfer or racquet sport enthusiast, avoid blisters on your hands by wearing gloves and keeping your hands and the grip dry. With new shoes or new equipment or a new season, take time to let your body develop calluses to protect potential points of irritation.

What can be done about skin irritation caused by clothing rubbing against the skin during exercise? The most common sites for exercise irritation are the armpits, crotch, thighs, and nipples. Liberal applications of petroleum jelly or similar substances may be helpful in both preventing and treating it.

How can athlete's foot and "jock itch" be treated? A good preventive measure for both "jock itch" and athlete's foot is to keep the vulnerable areas dry with talcum powder and by wearing dry, clean underclothing and socks. The powder absorbs sweat, which encourages fungal growth. If attention to hygiene doesn't help, try over-the-counter products containing either undecylenic acid or tolnaftate. Both are safe and effective antifungal remedies. If the infection persists, check with your physician or consult a podiatrist.

What can be done about a painful heel? It depends on the cause. If the pain is caused by Achilles tendinitis (inflammation of the Achilles tendon), it's a condition experienced by many joggers. The symptoms can vary from mild discomfort following exercise to total inability to walk without severe pain. The Achilles tendon, which makes it possible to stand on one's toes, connects the calf muscle to the heel bone. Since it is richly supplied with nerve endings, it becomes very painful when inflamed. Tendinitis is most often caused by overuse. Moderate stress on a tendon may result in microscopic tears. With greater stress, the tendon may rupture or break entirely, requiring surgical repair.

Ideally, tendinitis should be treated with rest. Discontinue jogging, cut down on walking, and try to stay off the foot as much as possible. But go on stretching out your heels and ankles gently every day. You can continue to maintain fitness by substituting swimming or bicycling for the duration. When you feel well enough to resume running, begin at a reduced intensity, duration, and frequency. Gradually build up your exercise program, if there is no recurrence of your tendon problem.

If the condition is mild enough to allow you to continue running, you should reduce the intensity, duration, and frequency. Joggers, for instance, can alternate running with walking as a temporary measure. Be sure to stretch well and warm up thoroughly. (See the stretching model program in Chapter 7.)

Some people find it helpful to apply heat to the calf before stretching, or to massage it with ice afterward. Check your running shoes. Running in shoes with badly rundown heels can cause tendinitis. Try wearing shoes with built-up heels to reduce the strain, or try putting felt heel pads in your shoes.

If you're a beginning jogger, you can try to prevent tendon problems by keeping off hard surfaces, if possible, until you have developed good flexibility of the legs and until you are sure you have the best possible footwear and heel padding. Be sure you are running so that your heel strikes the ground first (or at least the whole foot). Never run so that your full weight is on the ball of the foot.

To strengthen the antagonistic muscles—those muscles around the shin that work in opposition to the calf muscles—try walking on your heels or raising your foot toward your shin while pressing down on your toes, for example. There is a tendency among runners to ignore the shin muscles while the calf muscles become very strong. The result is an imbalance that can complicate the problem of tendinitis. A series of simple strengthening exercises can help balance out the musculature of the lower leg and foot and thus help prevent future episodes of pain.

If the problem persists, you may want to consult an orthopedist, a podiatrist, or a physical therapist specializing in sports injuries. Be sure that such a person has had experience with this sort of condition. Many times, a device called an orthotic (see below) can be inserted in your running shoes. If this does not help, you may have to reconsider your exercise program. Some people have legs and feet that simply cannot stand up to the punishment that running demands. If you are one of them, choose another form of cardiorespiratory endurance (CRE) training from CRE activities described in Chapter 3 or in Chapter 7.

What about orthotics? In the March 1981 *Consumer Reports,* orthotics for runners were discussed. A fancier version of an arch support, an orthotic is an individually molded insole. The magazine reported as follows:

"Custom-made orthotics can be expensive. In the New York area, the cost for a pair is about $200. That includes X rays, a foot examination including 'gait analysis,' a plaster-of-paris mold of the feet, the orthotics made from the mold, and two or three follow-up office visits.

"Orthopedists agree that orthotics are useful in certain cases, but oppose widespread and indiscriminate use. They say there are other methods to redistribute the weight on the foot—methods that are much cheaper than using custom-made orthotics and just as effective. For many runners, the solution is to buy another brand of running shoes, one that will shift the weight-bearing areas of the foot, or to alternate two different pairs.

"We were not able to find any clear-cut scientific evidence that custom-made orthotics are more effective than the less expensive alternatives. If you've been told you need orthotics, our orthopedic consultants recommend that you first try one of the following products. If they don't work, you won't have harmed your feet.

■ Ready-made arch supports, which are available in various sizes.

■ Scaphoid pads, also known as 'cookies.' Firm, hard-rubber scaphoid pads are sold in most shoe stores and should provide better support than the soft latex pads that are built into the arch of many running shoes.

■ Inner heel wedges. These slanted wedges have long been used to correct pronation by tilting the heel outward. They're usually three-sixteenths of an inch high and are available at shoe-repair stores for about $8 to $10, installed."

What causes "backpacker's knee," and what can be done for it? Pain under the patella (kneecap)—variously called backpacker's, runner's, tennis, or jumper's knee—occurs when the patella does not ride in its proper groove as it moves over the knee joint. The friction may wear down the underside of the patella, causing inflammation and pain. Several abnormalities of gait can contribute to this problem. If, while running, your weight tends persistently to fall on the inside of your foot—a position called pronation—the turning and twisting of the leg bones may gradually make the patella unstable. Twisting may be the result of running on hard uneven surfaces, or of running in shoes that have worn down unevenly around the heels. The relative weakness of the quadriceps muscles (on the front of the thighs) compared with the strength of the hamstring muscles (on the back of the thighs) creates an imbalance that affects the pull of the muscles on the patella, thus irritating the joint. Less frequently, a runner with legs of unequal length may develop pelvic tilting that, again, may result in twisting of the knee.

If you suffer from backpacker's knee, try applying ice to the painful area as soon as possible. To correct some of the underlying difficulties, see the exercises for the knee in the Glossary of Exercises to strengthen the quadriceps and to stretch the hamstrings. This combination of exercises is designed to counteract any imbalance that may be affecting the patella. Be sure you use good, well-fitting shoes with a solid shank and an adequate, supporting heel counter. If the problem persists, consult an orthopedist or a podiatrist.

Sometimes the pain of backpacker's knee is so severe that you should keep all weight off the affected leg and give it a period of rest. Try switching to swimming or cycling until you can return to running, hiking, or tennis again.

What causes "tennis elbow" and what can be done for it? Tennis elbow can be disabling. An inflammation of tendons that link the forearm muscles to the elbow, it is caused by an overload of pressure on the forearm muscle groups that results in straining of the tendons at the elbow. While the problem is called tennis elbow, probably because it is so common among tennis players, it occurs in all racquet, wall, and net sports (as well as among gardeners, carpenters, lumberjacks, and house-cleaners). Authorities have identified the following as contributing to tennis elbow: using the forearm as the source of power rather than body weight transferred from the shoulder; hitting a ball off-center on a racquet; using a racquet that is too heavy, has too large a grip, or has too much tension on the strings; playing on a surface that produces a greater velocity of speed to the ball and results in a greater force being trans-mitted to the forearm and elbow. Treatment of tennis elbow may require medical attention. Start a program to increase the strength, endurance, and flexibility of the arm and shoulder after the pain subsides.

As a preventive measure, try improving your stroking ability to make contact with the ball properly—by using body weight coming from the shoulder as the source of power. A two-handed grip to hit a backhand can also be useful. Proper warm-up, particularly easy stretching of the elbow and its surrounding tissue, is essential.

What are shinsplints, and what can be done about it? Shinsplints is a term used for a variety of conditions that produce pain along the front of the lower leg, that is, over the shinbone (tibia). It is often caused by an imbalance between a strengthened and shortened calf muscle and a comparatively weak shin muscle—a frequent result of prolonged strenu-ous running or jumping, particularly on hard surfaces. The pain itself may be the result of microscopic stress fractures of the tibia, a reduced blood supply to the muscles attached to the tibia, or damage from over-stretching or overloading the muscles and tendons surrounding the tibia.

The best way to relieve the pain of shinsplints is to rest with the leg elevated and apply an ice pack to the painful area. To improve the condition, try wearing shoes with a raised heel or extra padding to absorb shock. Avoid exercising on hard surfaces. To strengthen the shin muscles and to stretch the calf muscles, refer to the Glossary of Exercises. Reduce the intensity and duration of your activity, and avoid running uphill until the condition improves. If these measures fail, consult an orthopedist, a podiatrist, or a physical therapist who is familiar with runners' problems. You may need to have an orthotic designed and molded especially to fit into your shoe to correct your gait.

What are stress fractures? Stress fractures are hairline cracks in a bone. They occur most commonly in the bones of the lower leg and foot. The pain of a stress fracture is similar to that of shinsplints, except that it is much more sharply localized. Diagnosis is usually confirmed by X ray, although sometimes a stress fracture shows up only some weeks after it has occurred, when callus formation becomes visible. You may be able to continue exercising with a stress fracture, but at reduced levels of intensity and duration. In more severe cases, you may have to stay off your feet entirely for several weeks. To prevent recurrence, do the exercises for the foot and ankle in the Glossary of Exercises. If stress fractures persist, you may need to consider changing to an activity that requires less impact on your feet, such as swimming or cycling.

What can be done about sprained ankles? A sprained ankle is a common complaint, especially among joggers and runners. A sprain is an injury to the ligaments that surround a joint and help keep it stable. It may be a slight stretching of the ligaments or it may consist of a number of small tears. If you don't give the ligaments enough time to heal completely before you resume your activity, your ankle may be susceptible to further injury. The best way to treat a sprain is to elevate it and apply ice as soon possible. You may use an elastic bandage for support—psychological as well as physical—and a cane or crutches if the pain is severe. When the pain subsides and any swelling has gone down, you may begin to rehabilitate the ankle. Do the exercises for the foot and ankle in the Glossary of Exercises to strengthen the muscles of the ankle and maintain flexibility. When you return to your regular exercise program, be sure to protect your weak ankle until it gets stronger. Your shoes should fit well and have well-cushioned soles. Avoid running on uneven surfaces. Above all, watch out for potholes, roots, stones, curbs, and other stumbling blocks.

Does jogging only on Saturdays and Sundays do more harm than good? Although weekend jogging does not satisfy the recommended three days a week of CRE exercise (see Chapter 3), it can, of course, do some good. If you jog regularly every weekend, you will experience some improvement in CRE. The only way it can do you harm is if you try to make up for lost time by working out too strenuously on Saturdays and Sundays. Keep the intensity of your run within your exercise benefit zone (see pages 62–66), and keep the duration within comfortable bounds. If you don't push yourself too close to the limits of your muscular and skeletal systems, you should be able to avoid pain and injury.

How do you maintain fitness once you achieve your goals? Once you achieve the fitness goals you've set for yourself, you can then set higher ones, or decide to go on a maintenance program to keep yourself at goal levels. Generally, maintenance requires somewhat less effort. You can reduce frequency, but you should stick with the same intensity and duration. Continue to keep your progress chart, however. If you begin to notice a drop in fitness, you should increase intensity, duration, and frequency to return to goal levels.

Does sexual intercourse take away from athletic performance? Not at all. The notion that athletes would be well advised to keep away from all sexual activity while in training and certainly before an event is pure myth. Any moderately conditioned individual should recover very quickly from burning the limited number of calories used in intercourse (ranging from as few as it takes to wash or dress to at most a brisk walk). In fact, orgasm induces a state of relaxation and for some a desire to rest or sleep. This should not be confused with fatigue. Some athletes report that sexual activity helps to relieve some of the unproductive tension often experienced before an athletic event.

Do physically fit people have a better sex life than other people? No one knows. There is, however, no shortage of theory on this subject. No carefully controlled studies have been carried out to determine if there is a measurable, consistent relationship between physical fitness and one's sex life. Many people who exercise regularly—including many of the *Consumer Reports* readers who wrote to us about their exercise experience —do report that increased enjoyment of sexual activity is a major benefit of their athletic activity.

Do people become addicted to exercise? Some exercisers, particularly runners, do seem to become addicted to the sport. They give their daily run top priority, convinced that they cannot survive without it. They run despite pain, illness, or injury, putting their all-consuming passion for the sport ahead of family, job, and health. Some runners may even suffer withdrawal symptoms if forced to stop running. They become anxious, irritable, or depressed; they may get tics, muscle spasms, loss of appetite, constipation, and insomnia. Whether this extreme kind of dependency is based on physiological or psychological causes (or both) is not known.

Is Cooper's aerobics system useful? Kenneth Cooper, M.D., asserts that the regular performance of vigorous aerobic exercise builds cardio-respiratory fitness. According to Cooper, by doing such things as walking, swimming, or playing tennis or squash at high intensity for specified durations and frequencies, you can improve the condition of your lungs, heart, and blood vessels. Furthermore, according to Cooper, you can

261

improve your chances of avoiding coronary heart disease, hypertension, varicose veins, stomach ulcers, diabetes, obesity, back pain, arthritis, glaucoma, insomnia, and depression. With his books and articles and his appearances on television, Cooper has made the American public familiar with his system of aerobics.

Central to Cooper's system is the "point scale" that serves as a guide to weekly exercise goals. Every point in Cooper's system represents seven milliliters of oxygen consumed per minute per kilogram of body weight. This means that if you walk one mile in twenty minutes, for example, you earn one point. Do this five times a week, and you get five points. According to Cooper, if you walk three miles in forty-three minutes and thirty seconds, five times a week, you get forty points. Cooper recommends that you average thirty to thirty-two points per week to maintain cardiorespiratory endurance and cardiac health.

As cardiorespiratory conditioning, Cooper's aerobics system has many advantages. It allows you to exercise within your exercise benefit zone for a minimum of fifteen minutes for each workout. The point scales are simple and easy to use. Progress is easily measured. There are clear weekly goals, and a wide choice of activities.

Cooper's system, however, focuses almost entirely on CRE. He recommends dietary control along with an aerobic exercise program to control weight or reduce body fat, but he makes few recommendations regarding flexibility or muscular strength and endurance. If you follow Cooper's aerobic system, you should supplement it with strengthening and stretching exercises for a more balanced program.

What happens if you don't do any exercise at all? After twenty-eight days in space, the three astronauts of Skylab I returned to earth so weak that they couldn't stand without support. Their physicians were alarmed, especially when the weakness persisted. The astronauts' cardiorespiratory fitness had evidently deteriorated during their four weeks of sedentary living outside the pull of the earth's gravity. Learning from that experience, planners at the National Aeronautics and Space Administration installed exercise equipment—a stationary bicycle in Skylab II and both a bike and a treadmill in Skylab III. As a result, the astronauts of Skylabs II and III, who remained in space two and three times as long as the men of Skylab I, returned to earth with very little loss of fitness.

Of course, the most sedentary person on earth has fewer problems than an astronaut in space, who does not have even the pull of gravity to work against. But an earthbound person who sits in a chair long enough may become capable of doing little else but sit in a chair. Almost any physical effort would be exhausting for the totally sedentary person. Because the body adapts in time to whatever load is regularly placed upon it, the ability to work is reduced if the load lessens.

Glossary of Exercises
Appendixes

Glossary of Exercises

There are literally thousands of different exercises to be performed with or without equipment. There are limitless combinations of exercises possible to meet virtually every individual need. The exercises selected for this Glossary should provide enough variety for most exercisers.

Each exercise is named so it can be readily recognized. Each is also numbered, to help you locate the exercise as easily as possible. The body parts affected by each exercise is also noted following the name of the exercise. The instructions are brief but adequate. Use the illustrations to assist you in fully understanding the exercise. And take special care to note the safety hints found in the instructions of many of the exercises.

The Glossary is divided into two parts: exercises that require equipment and exercises that do not require equipment. The first part has five sections: barbell exercises (1B through 23B); cable exercises (1C through 5C); dumbbell exercises (1D through 8D); lever exercises (1L through 3L); and exercises that require machines (1M through 4M). The second part has three sections: calisthenic exercises (1E through 26E); flexibility exercises (1F through 22F); and aqua exercises (1Q through 6Q).

Exercises for the major joints

The following list of exercises involve the major joints: shoulder, elbow, wrist, knee, and foot and ankle. They can be used by people who have arthritic problems or orthopedic difficulties, or who wish to strengthen or stretch the muscles of a major joint.

Shoulder	Elbow	Knee
1B, 2B, 5B, 22B	5B, 7B, 8B, 11B, 12B, 22B	15B, 17B, 19B,
1C		2M, 3M, 4M
1D, 2D, 3D, 4D	2C, 4C, 5C	9E, 10E, 23E, 26E
1M	2D, 7D	2F, 3F, 10F, 11F
2E	25E, 26E	**Foot and ankle**
18F, 19F, 20F, 21F, 22F	**Wrist**	19B
	9B, 10B	14F, 15F
	1L, 2L, 3L	

Barbell exercises

The barbell is a piece of adjustable weight training equipment that requires both hands.

1B. Shoulder shrug (neck, shoulders)

Raise and lower your shoulders, keeping your arms straight. Try to touch your ears with your shoulders.

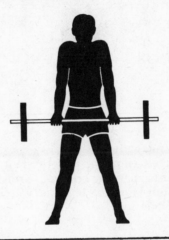

2B. Upright rowing (shoulders, upper back, arms)

Lift the barbell to your chin, keeping your elbows high.

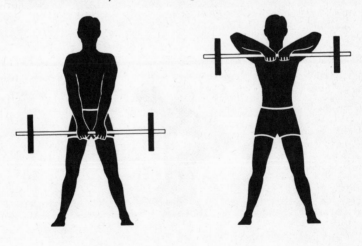

265

3B. Bent rowing (upper back, arms)

With your back flat and knees bent, raise the barbell to your chest, keeping your elbows high.

Safety. Do this exercise while resting your head on a table.

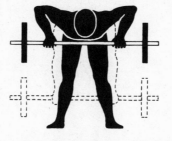

4B. Clean and press (full body)

Lift the barbell from the floor to your chest in one movement and then push it over your head, using only your arms.

Safety. Be sure your knees are bent and your back is flat when lifting the barbell from the floor.

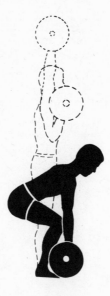

5B. Military press (upper back, shoulders, arms)

From your shoulders push the barbell over your head, using only your arms.

Safety. Push the barbell directly or slightly backward over your head so that it is in line with the center of gravity.

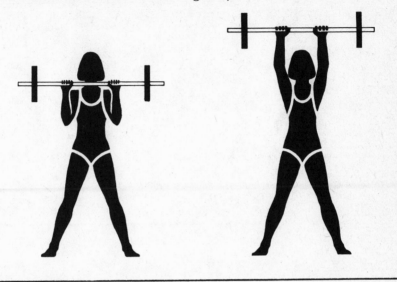

6B. Behind-the-neck press (upper back, shoulders, arms)

From the back of your neck push the barbell overhead, using only your arms.

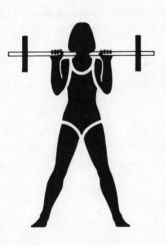
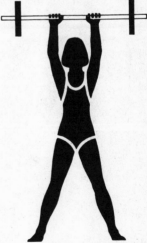

7B. Curl (biceps, forearms)

With your palms forward and elbows close to your sides, bend your elbows, bringing the barbell up to your chest. Do not swing your body forward and back. Maintain a stationary position.

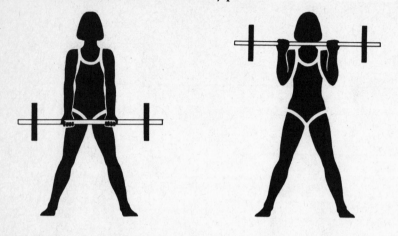

8B. Reverse curl (biceps, forearms)

Same as curl (7B), except your knuckles are forward instead of your palms.

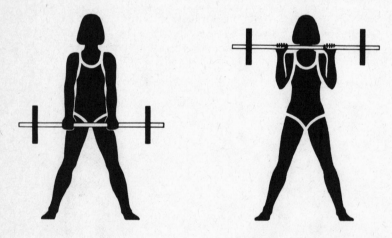

9B. Regular wrist curl (wrists, forearms)

Sit down and rest your forearms on your thighs. Grasp the barbell with your palms forward and curl the barbell up toward your forearms.

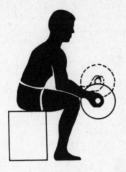

10B. Reverse wrist curl (wrists, forearms)

Same as regular wrist curl (9B), except your knuckles are forward instead of your palms.

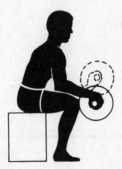

11B. Standing triceps press (triceps)

Lower the barbell from over your head, keeping your elbows pointed forward and toward the ceiling and your arms close to your ears. Then straighten your elbows while maintaining the vertical position of the upper arms.

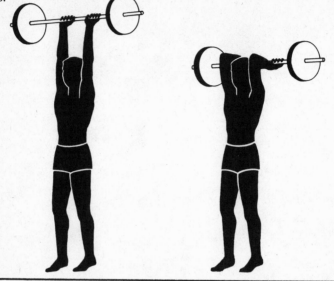

12B. Supine triceps press (triceps)

Lower the barbell to the bridge of your nose, keeping your elbows pointed forward and toward the ceiling. Then straighten your elbows while maintaining the vertical position of the upper arms.

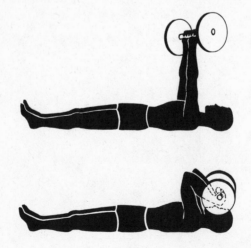

13B. Bend-over (lower back, hips, hamstrings)

With the barbell on the back of your shoulders, bend forward until your trunk is in a horizontal position, keeping your head up. Return to upright position.

Safety. Avoid this exercise if you have serious back problems.

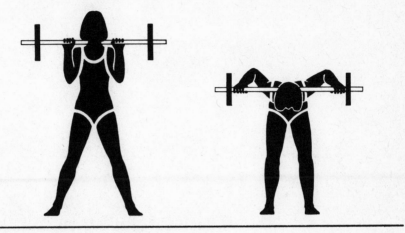

14B. Regular dead lift (lower back, thighs)

Squat to grasp the barbell, which is at your front, and lift it by straightening your knees until you come to a standing position.

Safety. Always bend the knees, keep the back flat, and head up when lifting a weight from the floor and when returning it to the floor.

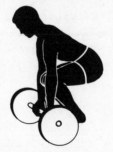

15B. Hack lift (hips, lower back)

Squat and grasp the barbell, which is behind you, and lift it by straightening your knees until you come to a standing position.

Safety. Always bend the knees, keep the back flat, and head up when lifting a weight from the floor and when returning it to the floor.

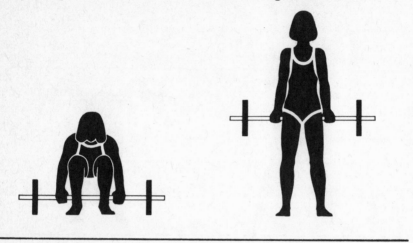

16B. Straddle lift (thighs)

Squat and grasp the barbell, which is between your feet, and lift it by straightening your knees until you come to a standing position. Note that the front hand has the palm forward and the back hand has the knuckles forward.

Safety. Always bend the knees, keep the back flat, and head up when lifting a weight from the floor and when returning it to the floor.

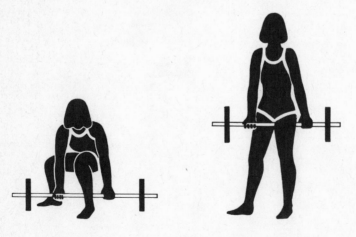

17B. Parallel squat (quadriceps, hips)

With the barbell resting on the back of your shoulders, lower your body by bending at the knees. In the squat position the top of your thighs should be parallel with the floor.

Safety. To prevent squatting below the parallel level, you may wish to touch your buttocks to a chair or bench. Keep your back flat and head up.

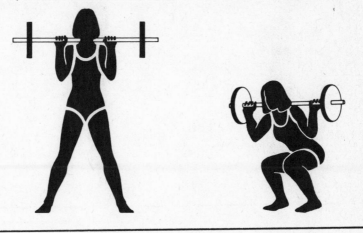

18B. Jumping squat (thighs, hips, buttocks, lower legs)

Lower your body to a parallel squat as in exercise 17B and then jump as high as possible, straightening your knees and pushing downward with the toes so that you leave the floor.

Safety. Land with your knees slightly bent to absorb shock. See safety precautions for parallel squat (17B).

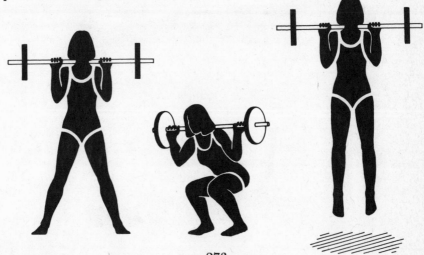

19B. Raise on toes (lower legs)

With the barbell resting on the back of your shoulders, stand with the balls of your feet on a two-inch board. Raise your heels from the floor and return.

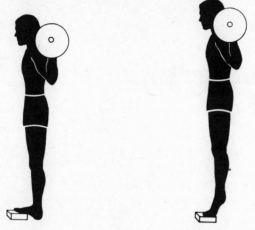

20B. Straight arm pull-over (chest, upper back)

Keeping your arms straight, bring the barbell above your chest in a forward movement, and then return it *slowly* to the floor.

Safety. Control the weight so that it doesn't strike your face.

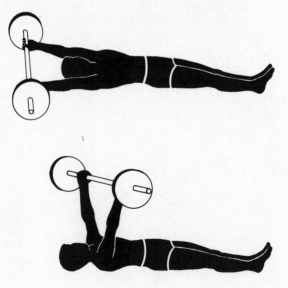

21B. Bent arm pull-over (chest, upper back)

Keeping your elbows bent, pull the bar directly to a resting position on your chest, and then return it *slowly* to the floor.

Safety. Control the weight so that it doesn't strike your face.

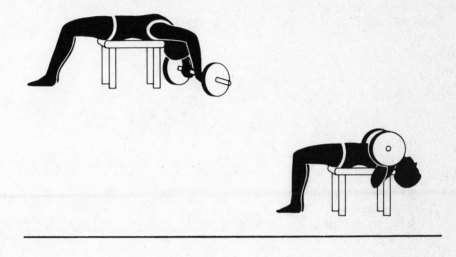

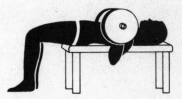

22B. Bench press (chest, triceps)

Grasp the bar with your palms forward and your hands as wide apart as possible. Lower the barbell to your chest and then push it back to the starting position.

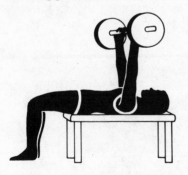

23B. Bent arm pull-over and press (upper back, chest, triceps)

This is a combination of exercises 21B and 22B. Read the instructions and safety precautions for these two exercises.

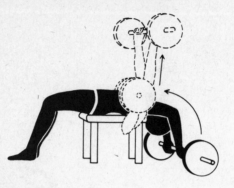

Cable exercises

Some dumbbell exercises can be performed using cables. Here, however, are several exercises unique to cables (also known as the spring exerciser).

Safety. Perform all cable exercises slowly and under control so that the cables do not snap back.

1C. Front pull (upper back, shoulders)

With your arms straight out in front of you, slowly stretch the cables horizontally to the side until they touch your chest. Return *slowly* to the starting position.

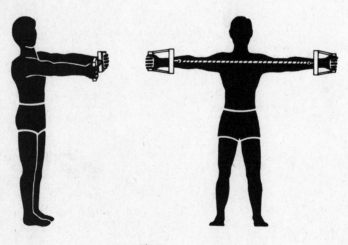

2C. Archer's exercise (upper back, triceps)

Keeping one arm straight, extend the other arm at the elbow horizontally to the side; alternate these movements.

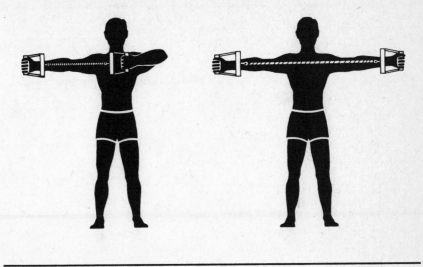

3C. Overhead pull (upper back, chest)

With your arms up and diagonally outward, pull your arms horizontally downward to the side until the cables touch the front of your chest. Palms can be inward or outward.

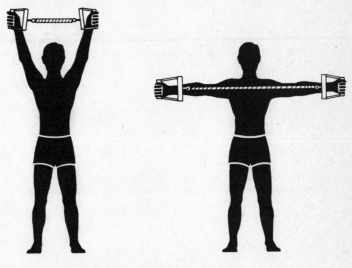

4C. Front press (triceps, upper back)

   With your elbows bent, knuckles on the outside, and the cables held in front of your shoulders, press your arms straight out to the side until the cables touch your chest. Return *slowly* to the starting position.

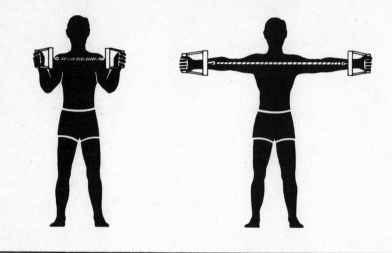

5C. Back press (triceps)

   Same as front press (4C), except the cables are behind your back.

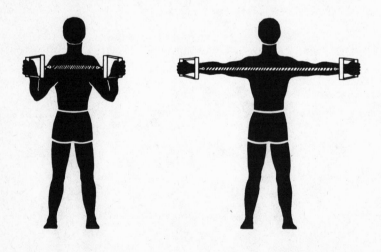

Dumbbell exercises

Dumbbells usually come in pairs. They also come in a variety of weights and designs.

1D. Lateral raise (shoulders)

With your knuckles facing out and up and your arms straight, raise the dumbbells to shoulder level and then return to the starting position.

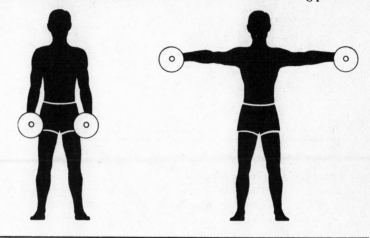

2D. Forward raise (shoulders, upper back)

With knuckles forward and your arms straight, raise both arms overhead and return to the starting position.

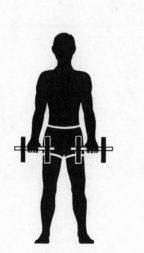
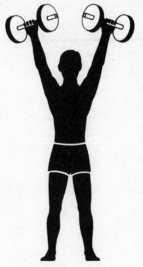

3D. Bend-over lateral raise (shoulders, upper back)

Start with your torso bent forward at a right angle. Raise the dumbbells sideward and upward with your knuckles toward the ceiling, and then lower to the starting position.

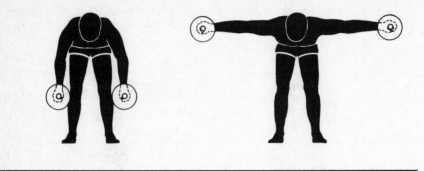

4D. Lateral raise, lying (chest)

Lower the dumbbells to your side below the level of the bench with your arms bent slightly at the elbows. Return to the starting position.

Safety. Restrict the distance that you lower the dumbbells until you're familiar with the exercise.

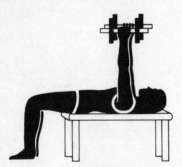

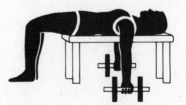

5D. Side bend (trunk)

Hold the dumbbell in one hand, palm in, arm straight. Place the other hand behind your head, keeping your elbow high. Bend the dumbbell side as far as you can without leaning forward. Alternate hands, and repeat on the other side.

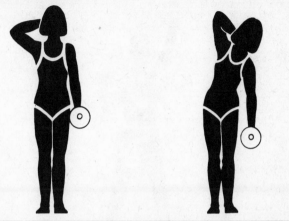

6D. Single dumbbell toe touch (trunk)

Bend over and touch your right foot with your left hand while holding the dumbbell over your head in your right hand. After a number of repetitions, repeat the exercise using the other hand to hold the dumbbell.

Safety. Use a light weight until you perfect the exercise, and bend your knees slightly until you can maintain straight knees without straining.

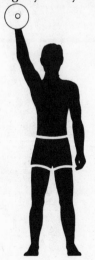
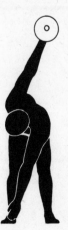

7D. Alternate press (shoulders, chest, upper back, triceps)

Lift the left dumbbell overhead, palm facing the body. As you lower the left dumbbell to the shoulder starting position, simultaneously lift the right dumbbell overhead: As one dumbbell is lowered, the other is lifted.

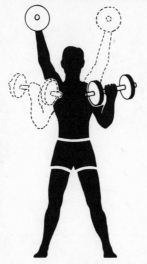

8D. Forward swing (thighs, lower back, shoulders, upper back)

Swing the dumbbell overhead as you straighten your legs from a squat position. Return to the starting position with your back flat, knees slightly bent, and head up.

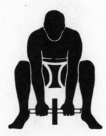 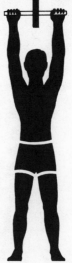

Lever exercises

The lever is an adjustable piece of weight training equipment that requires the use of one hand.

1L. Supination and pronation (wrist, forearm, biceps)

Keep your upper arm at your side and your forearm in a horizontal position. Hold the lever with palm up; rotate the lever overhand so your knuckles are up. Do not move the position of your arms.

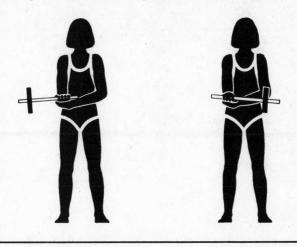

2L. Wrist lever forward (wrist, forearm)

Raise the lever forward using only your wrist, keeping your arm straight. Both arms remain at the side during the exercise.

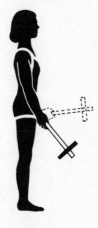

3L. Wrist lever backward (wrist, forearm)

Raise the lever to the rear by flexing the wrist, keeping your arm straight. Both arms remain at the side during this exercise. Do not let the weight sag.

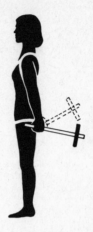

Exercises with machines

Many weight training exercises are performed using sophisticated equipment. If you exercise at a commercial or institutional facility, you will recognize these exercises.

1M. Pull-down (upper back, chest)

Pull the bar down to your chest and then slowly, and with control, return it to the starting position.

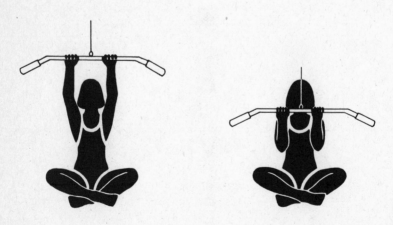

2M. Leg press (thighs, hips)
Push the pedal away from you by straightening your knees.

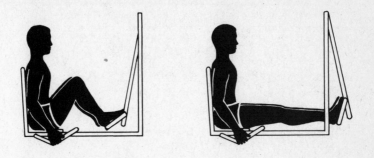

3M. Knee extension (quadriceps)
Pull the lever up by straightening your knees.

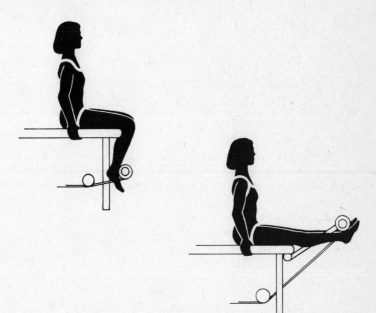

4M. Knee flexion (hamstrings)
Pull the lever up by bending your knees as far as possible.

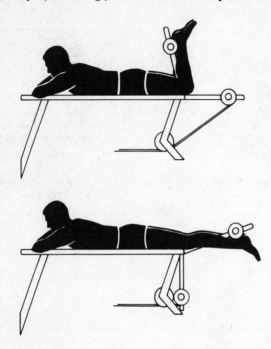

Calisthenic exercises

Calisthenic exercises are done without equipment. It is possible to perform many weight training exercises as calisthenic exercises simply by excluding the barbells or dumbbells.

1E. Neck circles (neck)
Rotate your neck forward to the right, to the rear, to the left, forward, and then reverse the rotation.

2E. Arm circles (shoulders)

Holding your arms sideward, palms up, circle forward and then reverse.

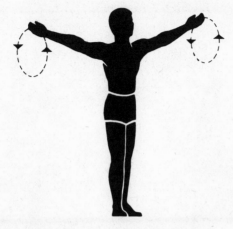

3E. Twister (hamstrings, trunk)

Bend forward with your back flat, your head up, and your knees straight. Twist your body to the left and then to the right. Touch first one foot and then the other. Keep your upper arm straight and over your back. (This can also be done with a wand or broomstick.)

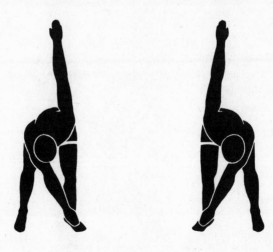

4E. Alternate toe touch (hamstrings, trunk)

Bend forward with your knees straight. Touch your right fingertips to your left foot and return to standing position. Bend forward with your knees straight. Touch your left fingertips to your right foot and return to standing position.

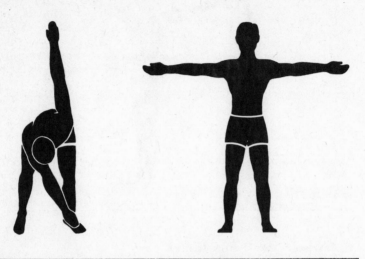

5E. Side bend (trunk)

Bend your body to the left (or right). Then reverse. Keep both hands behind your head.

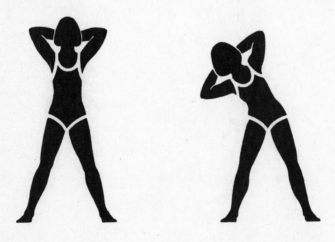

6E. Jumping jack (legs)

Start with your feet together, jump astride and clap your hands over your head. Then jump back to starting position.

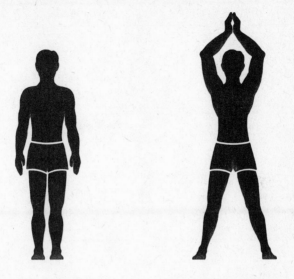

7E. Standing knee-to-chest (hips)

Raise first one knee and then the other, pulling the knee to your chest with your hands.

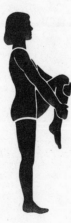

8E. Front kick (hips, quadriceps)

Kick your left (or right) foot forward as high as you can. Keep both legs straight. Hold on to something, if necessary.

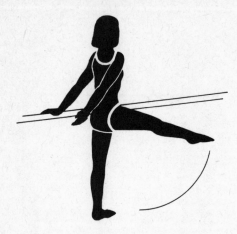

9E. Parallel squat (quadriceps, hips)

Keeping your back flat, bend your knees until the top of your thighs are parallel to the floor. Hold for two seconds and return to standing position.

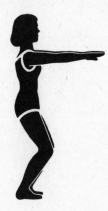

10E. Side lunge (quadriceps, legs, hips)

Lunge first to the right and then to the left, half squatting on the bent leg. Keep your extended leg straight.

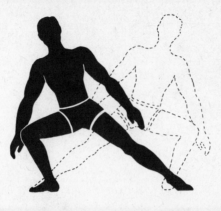

11E. Squat thrust (trunk, hips, thighs, arms)

From a standing position, squat and put your hands on the floor. Thrust both legs backward. Return to the squat position and stand before repeating the exercise.

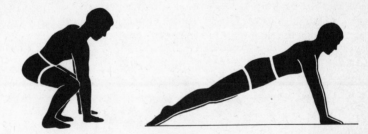

12E. Treadmill (trunk, hips, arms)

From a squat position, rhythmically extend first one leg and then the other backward, supporting yourself with your arms.

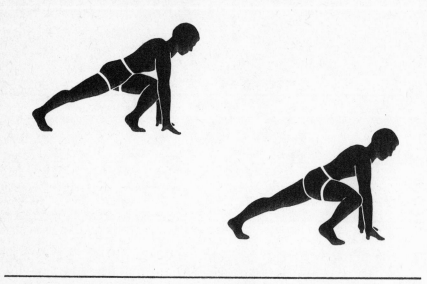

13E. Alternate knee-to-chest (abdominals, hips, lower back)

Bend one knee up to your chest; raise your head and try to touch your knee with your chin. Hold the bent leg with both hands at the knee. Alternate first one leg and then the other.

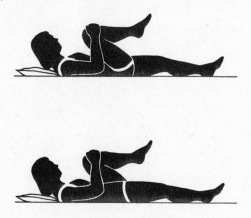

14E. Knee-to-chest (abdominals, hips, lower back)

Start with both feet flat on the floor. Bend both knees up to your chest. Keep your head down and your arms straight at your sides.

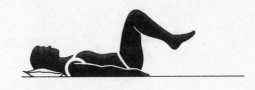

15E. Leg cross-overs (hips, back)

Raise one leg and cross it over your body. Keep your upper back flat and your arms extended to the sides. Alternate first one leg and then the other. Turn only your hips.

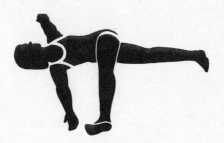

16E. Side leg raise (thighs, hips)

Raise one leg as high as possible, then return to starting position. Exercise first one side and then the other.

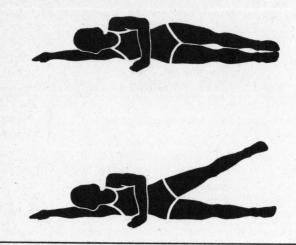

17E. Seated alternate knee-to-chest (hips, abdominals)

Raise first one knee and then the other up to your chest. As the bent leg is being returned to the floor, simultaneously bend the other knee up to your chest.

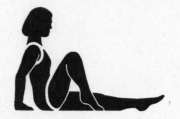

18E. Seated double knee-to-chest (hips, abdominals)

Same as seated alternate knee-to-chest (17E), except bend both knees to your chest.

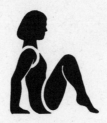

19E. Shoulder bridge (lower back)

Supporting your body on your feet and shoulders, raise your abdomen. Keep both hands behind your head or at your sides and your knees bent.

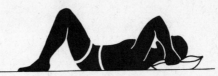

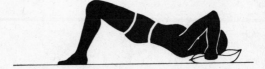

20E. Back extension (lower back)

Raise your head and shoulders. Keep your legs straight and your hands behind your head.

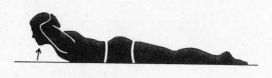

21E. Alternate hip extension (buttocks, hamstrings, lower back)

Raise first one leg and then the other as high as possible. Keep your legs straight and your hands clasped behind your back.

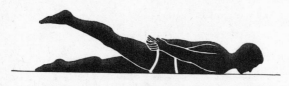

22E. One-leg mule kick (buttocks, hamstrings, hips)

Kick one leg and then the other back. Return your knee to your chest.

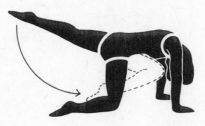

23E. Step-up (thighs, hips)

Step up with first one foot and then the other, alternating rhythmically up and down. As one foot goes up, the other comes down.

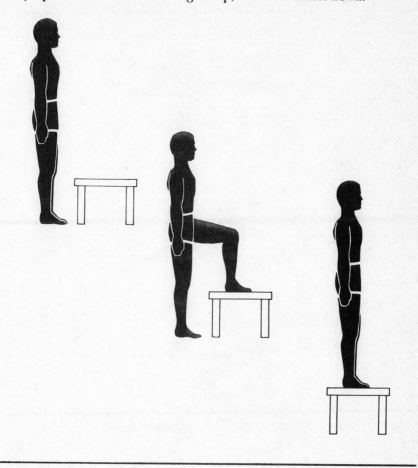

24E. Sit-up (abdominals)

There are several ways to perform the sit-up. The easiest way is to use your arms to help push your upper body into the sitting position. Next, you can thrust your arms directly out in front of you while sitting up. Or, if your abdominals are in fairly good shape, you can fold your arms across your chest. The most difficult position for the sit-up is placing your hands behind your head. If you use a slant board and can't do even one sit-up, start with your head at the high end of the board. As the sit-ups become easier, gradually lower the head of the board until you are doing sit-ups on a level surface. You can increase resistance by doing your sit-ups with your head at the lower end of the slant board. Always perform these exercises with your knees bent.

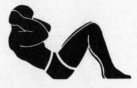

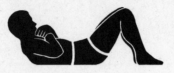

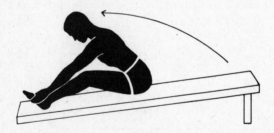

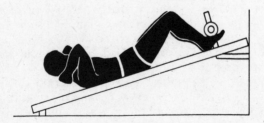

25E. Push-up (chest, triceps, upper back)

There are several ways to perform push-ups. The easiest way is to do them against a wall. Stand a straight-arm's distance away from the wall. Keeping your back and legs straight and your heels on the floor, lean forward until your nose touches the wall. Push your body back into a vertical position. Then there is the elevated push-up: First use a table (in place of the wall), then a chair, then an object lower than a chair—say, a box or a footstool. Try these variations, if the traditional floor position is difficult for you. To add resistance, raise your feet and then lower your chest to the floor.

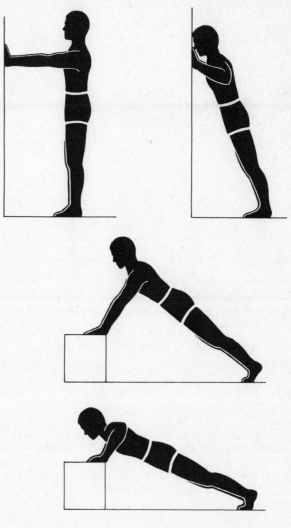

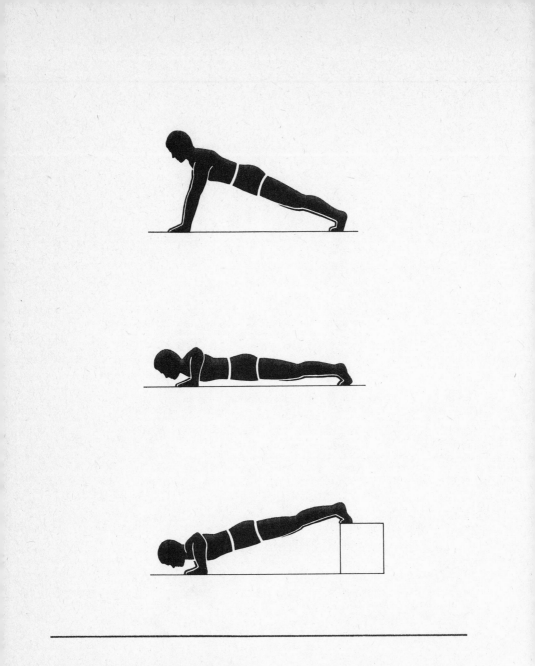

26E. Chin (upper back, chest, biceps)

Hang from an overhead bar with your arms straight. Bend your arms, pulling your body up until your chin is raised above the bar. This exercise can be difficult for some people. To work up to a chin, try lying down and, keeping your back and legs straight, pull your upper body up to the bar (which can be attached to the back of a chair or other support). Hold your chin above the bar as long as you can and lower yourself slowly.

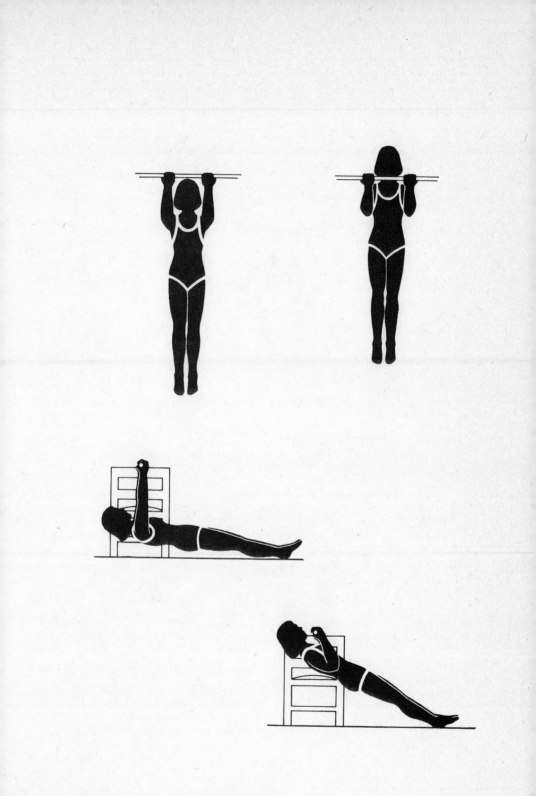

Flexibility exercises

In this section, stretching exercises for flexibility have been categorized according to the parts of the body involved.

1F. Standing toe touch (hamstrings)

Bend forward, reaching gradually for your toes. *Don't bounce.* Keep your knees straight and your head down. Eventually you will be able to place your palms on the floor.

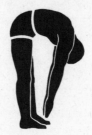

2F. Leg rest on chair back (hamstrings)

Rest one heel on a chair back or other support. Keep your knee straight and reach forward for your toes. Keep your head down.

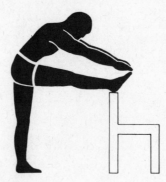

3F. Seated toe touch no. 1 (hamstrings)

Sit with your legs straight and gradually reach for your toes. Eventually you will be able to grasp your feet at the instep. Keep your head down.

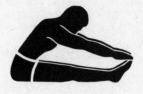

4F. Seated toe touch no. 2 (hamstrings)

Same as seated toe touch no. 1 (3F), except fold one leg in front.

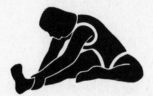

5F. Alternate knee-to-chest (lower back)

Bring one knee up to your chest. Curl your head toward your knee. Keep the other leg on the floor.

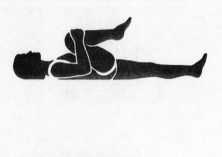

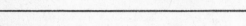

6F. Double knee-to-chest (lower back)

Same as alternate knee-to-chest (5F), except bring both knees up to your chest.

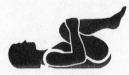

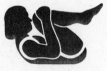

7F. Back-over (back, hamstrings)

Roll your legs over your head slowly. At first, allow your knees to bend and gradually progress to straight knees. Hold until you feel the stretch in your back. Position your arms as depicted, or where they are most comfortable for you.

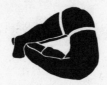

8F. Squat tuck (back)

Squat and curl yourself into a full-tuck position. Keep your hands clasped, head down, and heels on the floor. Hold this position until you feel the stretch in your back and thighs.

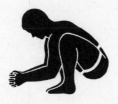

9F. Cat stretch on knees (upper back, shoulders)

Resting on your knees, reach forward with one arm and then the other to stretch your shoulders and back.

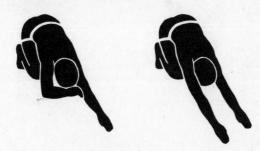

10F. Prone knee flexion (quadriceps)

Lying on your side with one arm tucked behind your head, use the other arm to slowly pull one foot up toward your buttocks. Flex the leg up until you feel the stretch in your quadriceps.

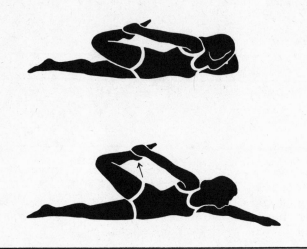

11F. Standing knee flexion (quadriceps)

Same as prone knee flexion (10F), except performed standing up. Use support to keep your balance, if necessary.

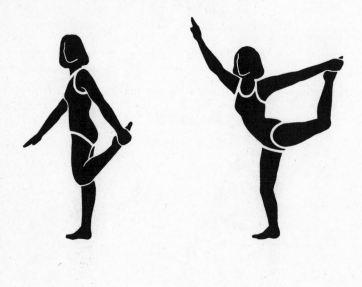

12F. Seated foot-over-knee twist (hips)

Seated as depicted, turn at the hips to face the rear. Hold your ankle to keep your foot on the floor. Alternate legs.

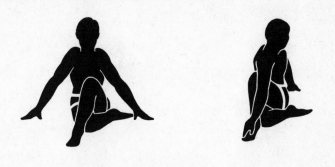

13F. Stride stretch (hips, hamstring)

Assume the racer's starting position and stretch one leg backward. Keep your head down. Alternate legs.

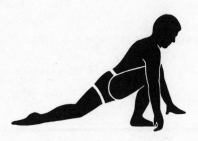

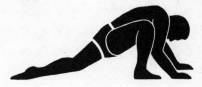

14F. Wall lean (lower legs)

Lean against the wall with one leg bent and the other straight. Keep your back straight and your heels on the floor. Bend the knee of the straight leg—this changes the stretch from the calf muscle to the Achilles tendon. Alternate legs.

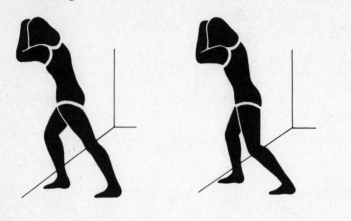

15F. Block stretch (lower legs)

Place the ball of one foot on a block, a step, or a curb. Keeping the leg straight, allow the heel to hang down over the edge to provide the stretch. Alternate legs.

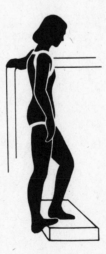

16F. Sole stretch (groin)

With the soles of your feet pressed together, pull your feet toward you while pressing your knees down with your elbows.

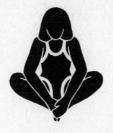

17F. Foot raise against wall (groin)

Rest one foot against a wall or other support. Lean forward, keeping your head down, and hands on the floor. Bending the supporting leg will increase the stretch.

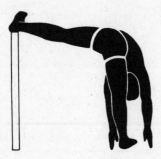

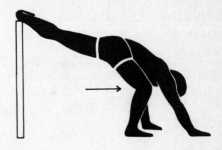

18F. Shoulder blade scratch (shoulders, arms)

Reach back with one arm as if to scratch your shoulder blade. Use your other hand to extend the stretch. Alternate arms.

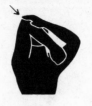

19F. Doorknob stretch (shoulders)

Holding on to a doorknob, bend forward extending your arms. Keep your legs straight. (Resting your weight on the doorknob will stretch your shoulders.)

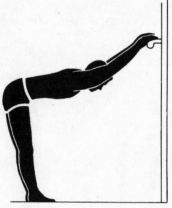

20F. Towel stretch (triceps, shoulders, upper back)

Grasp a rolled towel at both ends and slowly bring it back over your head as far down as possible. Keep your arms straight. (The closer your hands are, the greater the stretch.)

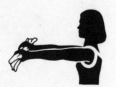 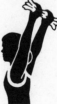

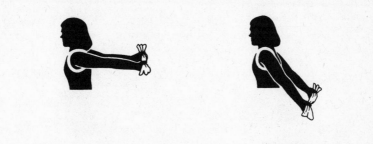

21F. Doorway stretch (chest, shoulders)

Hold the door jambs with your arms straight behind you. (Leaning forward will increase the stretch.)

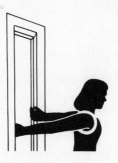

22F. Reach back (chest, shoulders)

While seated, inch backward with your hands. Keep your legs straight and your head up. (The farther back you can go, the greater the stretch.)

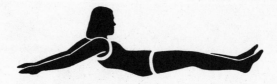

Aqua exercises

Aqua exercises require no equipment—just a pool to do them in.

1Q. Elementary bobbing (thighs)

Stand in shallow water, inhale, and duck underwater to a squat position while exhaling. Push off the pool bottom to a standing position and inhale.

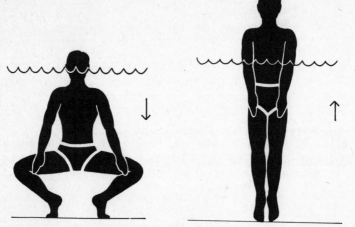

2Q. High bobbing (thighs, chest, upper back)

In water over your head, inhale and drop down to a squat position, keeping arms overhead. Exhale on the way down. Jump upward, thrusting your legs and pulling your arms down to your sides. Inhale at the peak of your jump.

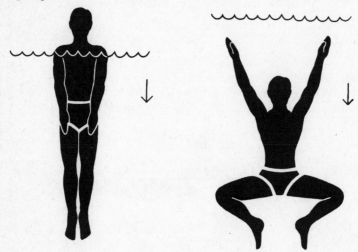

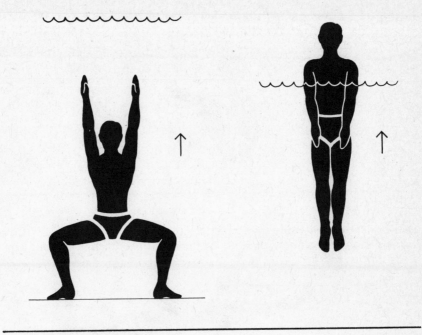

3Q. Elementary treading (arms, legs)

In water deep enough so your feet don't touch bottom, tread water by using your hands and feet. Scull or fin with your hands as you bicycle, scissor, or frog kick.

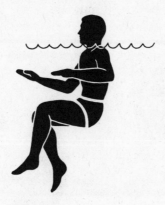

4Q. Climbing (arms, legs)
Hold on to the pool gutter and walk up and down the pool side.

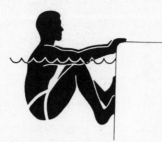

5Q. Front flutter kicking (quadriceps, hips)
Hold on to the pool side while lying on your stomach. Kick your legs, using a flutter kick.

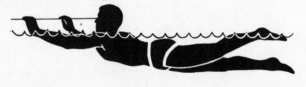

6Q. Pool-side knees up (abdominals, hips)
Hold on to the pool side while lying on your back. Bring your knees up to your chin and then extend your legs.

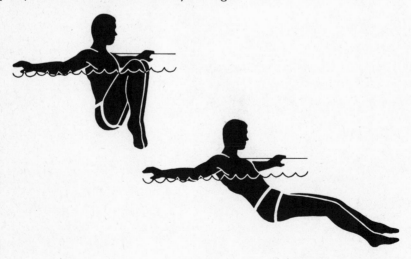

Appendixes

Appendix A

Estimating Oxygen Consumption

If your oxygen consumption score was not calculated at the time you took a cardiac stress test, you can still estimate your score. If you were tested on a treadmill, two bits of information are needed: the percent of grade (elevation) of the treadmill and your maximum speed of walking or running. (Use the percent of the grade and maximum speed achieved for at least 2 minutes.) Apply these to Table A–1 to get your oxygen consumption score.

If you were tested on a bicycle ergometer, you need your body weight and the work load at maximum heart rate. (Your work load may be available in kilopond-meters per minute or in watts.*) Apply these to Table A–2 to get your oxygen consumption score.

Once you have your oxygen consumption score, turn to Table 1–6, page 29, to get your rating.

---

*Kilopond-meter: Energy necessary to lift a 1-kilogram (2.2046 pounds) mass 1 meter (39.37 inches) against the normal gravitational force. Watt: A unit of power equal to 6.12 kilopond-meters per minute.

Table A–1

Estimating Oxygen Consumption with Treadmill Test

The Table below can be used to estimate oxygen consumption for a walking or running treadmill test for at least 2 minutes at maximum. Results are given in milliliters of oxygen consumption per kilogram of body weight per minute. For example: If you weigh 130 pounds, multiply 130 times .454 to get your body weight in kilograms (59 kilograms). Then, if you walked at 3 miles per hour on a 7.5 percent elevation, the result would be 21 (see Table) milliliters of oxygen per kilogram of body weight: $21 \times 59 = 1,239$ estimated milliliters of oxygen consumed. The same formula applies to running, below.

Percent of elevation	Speed of walking (miles per hour)							
	1.7	2.0	2.5	3.0	3.4	3.5	4.0	4.2
0.0	5.95	7.0	8.75	10.5	11.9	12.25	16.1	17.5
2.5	8.05	9.45	11.55	14.0	15.75	16.45	21.0	22.75
5.0	10.15	11.9	14.7	17.5	19.95	20.65	25.55	27.65
7.5	11.9	14.0	17.5	21.0	24.15	24.85	30.45	32.55
10.0	14.0	16.45	20.65	24.5	28.0	29.05	35.0	37.8
12.0	15.75	18.55	23.1	27.65	31.5	32.2	38.85	41.65
12.5	16.10	18.90	23.8	28.0	32.2	33.25	39.9	42.7
14.0	17.15	20.30	25.55	30.45	35.0	35.7	42.7	45.5
15.0	18.20	21.35	26.6	31.5	36.05	37.45	44.8	47.6
16.0	18.90	22.40	28.0	33.25	37.8	38.5	46.55	49.7
17.5	20.30	23.80	29.75	35.0	40.25	41.30	49.35	52.5
20.0	22.05	26.25	32.55	38.5	44.45	45.5	54.25	57.75

Percent of elevation	Speed of running (miles per hour)			
	6.0	7.0	8.0	9.0
0.0	35.0	40.25	44.8	49.7
2.5	39.9	44.45	49.35	53.9
5.0	44.45	49.0	53.9	58.45
7.5	48.65	53.55	58.1	63.0
10.0	53.20	57.75	62.65	67.55
12.5	57.75	62.3	67.2	71.75

Table A-2

Estimating Oxygen Consumption with Bicycle Ergometer

The Table below can be used to estimate oxygen consumption during a cardiac stress test using a bicycle ergometer for at least 2 minutes at maximum. If your body weight does not appear in the column at the left, you can readily approximate your score by interpolating your weight at the appropriate point. Work load figures are given for both kilopond-meters per minute (kpm/min) and watts. Results are given in milliliters of oxygen consumption per kilogram of body weight per minute. For example: If you weigh 132 pounds, multiply 132 times .454 to get your body weight in kilograms (60 kilograms). Then, if your work load maximum is 600 kilopond-meters per minute, the result would be 25.55 (see Table) milliliters of oxygen per kilogram of body weight: $25.55 \times 60 = 1,533$ estimated milliliters of oxygen consumed. The same formula applies to work load in watts.

Body weight (in pounds)	Kpm/min: Watts:						Work load maximum						
	75 12	150 25	300 50	450 75	600 100	750 125	900 150	1050 175	1200 200	1350 225	1500 250	1650 275	1800 300
88	10.50	14.00	21.00	28.00	35.00	42.00	49.00	56.00	63.00	70.00	77.00		
110	9,80	12.60	18.20	23.80	29.40	35.00	40.25	46.20	51.80	57.05	63.00	68.60	73.50
132	9.45	11.55	16.45	21.00	25.55	30.45	35.00	39.55	44.45	49.00	53.55	58.45	63.00
154	9.10	10.85	15.05	18.90	23.10	26.95	30.80	35.00	38.85	42.70	46.90	49.00	54.95
176	8.75	10.50	14.00	17.50	21.00	24.50	28.00	31.50	35.00	38.50	42.00	45.50	49.00
198	8.40	10.15	13.30	16.45	19.60	22.40	25.55	28.70	31.85	35.00	38.15	41.30	44.10
220	8.40	9.80	12.60	15.40	18.20	21.00	23.80	26.60	29.40	32.20	35.00	37.80	40.60
242	8.40	9.45	11.90	14.70	17.15	19.60	22.05	24.85	27.30	29.75	32.55	35.00	37.45
264	8.05	9.45	11.55	14.00	16.45	18.55	21.00	23.45	25.55	28.00	30.45	32.55	35.00

Appendix B

Desirable Weights for Men and Women

This Table lists weights in pounds for men and women, age twenty-five and over, in indoor clothing. Weights are given according to height, including 1-inch heels for men and 2-inch heels for women. Use Table 1–7 on page 30 to help you decide whether your build is small, medium, or large.

Height	Small frame	Medium frame	Large frame
Men			
5' 2"	112–120	118–129	126–141
3"	115–123	121–133	129–144
4"	118–126	124–136	132–148
5"	121–129	127–139	135–152
6"	124–133	130–143	138–156
7"	128–137	134–147	142–161
8"	132–141	138–152	147–166
9"	136–145	142–156	151–170
10"	140–150	146–160	155–174
11"	144–154	150–165	159–179
6' 0"	148–158	154–170	164–184
1"	152–162	158–175	168–189
2"	156–167	162–180	173–194
3"	160–171	167–185	178–199
4"	164–175	172–190	182–204
Women			
4'10"	92–98	96–107	104–119
11"	94–101	98–110	106–112
5' 0"	96–104	101–113	109–125
1"	99–107	104–116	112–128
2"	102–110	107–119	115–131
3"	105–113	110–122	118–134
4"	108–116	113–126	121–138
5"	111–119	116–130	125–142
6"	114–123	120–135	129–146
7"	118–127	124–139	133–150
8"	122–131	128–143	137–154
9"	126–135	132–147	141–158
10"	130–140	136–151	145–163
11"	134–144	140–155	149–168
6' 0"	138–148	144–159	153–173

Appendix C

Procedure for Estimating Female Body Fat Percentage

Tables 1–8 and 1–9 on pages 32 and 33 give you examples of how women between the ages of 17 and 26, and 27 and 50 can estimate their percentage of body fat. Follow the instructions appropriate for your age group. Take the measurements required, use the constants listed for each of the three measurements, perform the calculations, and you'll have your estimated percent of body fat.

Table C–1

Estimating Body Fat for Females 17 to 26

To estimate body fat percentage for females 17 to 26, take the following three measurements:

A. Abdomen (1 inch above umbilicus)_____

B. Right thigh (directly below buttocks)_____

C. Right forearm (arm straight forward, palm up)_____.

Use the lists below to convert the measurements (in inches) of abdomen, right thigh, and right forearm into constants A, B, and C. Then apply the following formula:

Constant A _____ + Constant B _____ − Constant C _____ − 19.6 = _____ percent of body fat.

Abdomen		Right thigh		Right forearm	
Inches	Constant A	Inches	Constant B	Inches	Constant C
20.00	26.74	14.00	29.13	6.00	25.86
20.25	27.07	14.25	29.65	6.25	26.94
20.50	27.41	14.50	30.17	6.50	28.02
20.75	27.74	14.75	30.69	6.75	29.10
21.00	28.07	15.00	31.21	7.00	30.17
21.25	28.41	15.25	31.73	7.25	31.25
21.50	28.74	15.50	32.25	7.50	32.33
21.75	29.08	15.75	32.77	7.75	33.41
22.00	29.41	16.00	33.29	8.00	34.48
22.25	29.74	16.25	33.81	8.25	35.56
22.50	30.08	16.50	34.33	8.50	36.64
22.75	30.41	16.75	34.85	8.75	37.72
23.00	30.75	17.00	35.37	9.00	38.79
23.25	31.08	17.25	35.89	9.25	39.87
23.50	31.42	17.50	36.41	9.50	40.95
23.75	31.75	17.75	36.93	9.75	42.03
24.00	32.08	18.00	37.45	10.00	43.10

Abdomen		Right thigh		Right forearm	
Inches	Constant A	Inches	Constant B	Inches	Constant C
24.25	32.42	18.25	37.97	10.25	44.18
24.50	32.75	18.50	38.49	10.50	45.26
24.75	33.09	18.75	39.01	10.75	46.34
25.00	33.42	19.00	39.53	11.00	47.41
25.25	33.76	19.25	40.05	11.25	48.49
25.50	34.09	19.50	40.37	11.50	49.57
25.75	34.42	19.75	41.09	11.75	50.63
26.00	34.76	20.00	41.61	12.00	51.73
26.25	35.09	20.25	42.13	12.25	52.30
26.50	35.43	20.50	42.65	12.50	53.88
26.75	35.76	20.75	43.17	12.75	54.96
27.00	36.10	21.00	43.69	13.00	56.04
27.25	36.43	21.25	44.21	13.25	57.11
27.50	36.76	21.50	44.73	13.50	58.19
27.75	37.10	21.75	45.25	13.75	59.27
28.00	37.43	22.00	45.77	14.00	60.35
28.25	37.77	22.25	46.29	14.25	61.42
28.50	38.10	22.50	46.81	14.50	62.50
28.75	38.43	22.75	47.33	14.75	63.58
29.00	38.77	23.00	47.85	15.00	64.66
29.25	39.10	23.25	48.37	15.25	65.73
29.50	39.44	23.50	48.89	15.50	66.81
29.75	39.77	23.75	49.41	15.75	67.89
30.00	40.11	24.00	49.93	16.00	68.97
30.25	40.44	24.25	50.45	16.25	70.04
30.50	40.77	24.50	50.97	16.50	71.12
30.75	41.11	24.75	51.49	16.75	72.20
31.00	41.44	25.00	52.01	17.00	73.28
31.25	41.78	25.25	52.53	17.25	74.36
31.50	42.11	25.50	53.05	17.50	75.43
31.75	42.45	25.75	53.57	17.75	76.51
32.00	42.78	26.00	54.09	18.00	77.39
32.25	43.11	26.25	54.61	18.25	78.67
32.50	43.45	26.50	55.13	18.50	79.74
32.75	43.78	26.75	55.65	18.75	80.82
33.00	44.12	27.00	56.17	19.00	81.90
33.25	44.45	27.25	56.69	19.25	82.98
33.50	44.78	27.50	57.21	19.50	84.05
33.75	45.12	27.75	57.73	19.75	85.13
34.00	45.45	28.00	58.26	20.00	86.21
34.25	45.79	28.25	58.78		
34.50	46.12	28.50	59.30		
34.75	46.46	28.75	59.82		
35.00	46.79	29.00	60.34		
35.25	47.12	29.25	60.86		
35.50	47.46	29.50	61.38		
35.75	47.79	29.75	61.90		
36.00	48.13	30.00	52.42		
36.25	48.46	30.25	62.42		
36.50	48.80	30.50	63.46		
36.75	49.13	30.75	63.98		
37.00	49.46	31.00	64.50		
37.25	49.80	31.25	65.02		
37.50	50.13	31.50	65.54		
37.75	50.47	31.75	66.06		

Abdomen		Right thigh	
Inches	Constant A	Inches	Constant B
38.00	50.80	32.00	66.58
38.25	51.13	32.25	67.10
38.50	51.47	32.50	67.62
38.75	51.80	32.75	68.14
39.00	52.14	33.00	68.66
39.25	52.47	33.25	69.18
39.50	52.81	33.50	69.70
39.75	53.14	33.75	70.22
40.00	53.47	34.00	70.74

Table C–2

Estimating Body Fat for Females 27 to 50

To estimate body fat percentage for females 27 to 50, take the following three measurements:

A. Abdomen (1 inch above umbilicus)_____

B. Right thigh (directly below buttocks)_____

C. Right calf (widest circumference midpoint between ankle and knee)_____.

Use the lists below to convert the measurements (in inches) of abdomen, right thigh, and right calf into constants A, B, and C. Then apply the following formula:

Constant A _____ + Constant B _____ − Constant C _____ − 18.4 = _____ percent of body fat.

Abdomen		Right thigh		Right calf	
Inches	Constant A	Inches	Constant B	Inches	Constant C
25.00	29.69	14.00	17.31	10.00	14.46
25.25	29.98	14.25	17.62	10.25	14.82
25.50	30.28	14.50	17.93	10.50	15.18
25.75	30.58	14.75	18.24	10.75	15.54
26.00	30.87	15.00	18.55	11.00	15.91
26.25	31.17	15.25	18.86	11.25	16.27
26.50	31.47	15.50	19.17	11.50	16.63
26.75	31.76	15.75	19.47	11.75	16.99
27.00	32.06	16.00	19.78	12.00	17.35
27.25	32.36	16.25	20.09	12.25	17.71
27.50	32.65	16.50	20.40	12.50	18.08
27.75	32.95	16.75	20.71	12.75	18.44
28.00	33.25	17.00	21.02	13.00	18.80
28.25	33.55	17.25	21.33	13.25	19.16
28.50	33.84	17.50	21.64	13.50	19.52
28.75	34.14	17.75	21.95	13.75	19.88

Abdomen		Right thigh		Right calf	
Inches	Constant A	Inches	Constant B	Inches	Constant C
29.00	34.44	18.00	22.26	14.00	20.24
29.25	34.73	18.25	22.57	14.25	20.61
29.50	35.03	18.50	22.87	14.50	20.97.
29.75	35.33	18.75	23.18	14.75	21.33
30.00	35.62	19.00	23.49	15.00	21.69
30.25	35.92	19.25	23.80	15.25	22.05
30.50	36.22	19.50	24.11	15.50	22.41
30.75	36.51	19.75	24.42	15.75	22.77
31.00	36.81	20.00	24.73	16.00	23.14
31.25	37.11	20.25	25.04	16.25	23.50
31.50	37.40	20.50	25.35	16.50	23.86
31.75	37.70	20.75	25.66	16.75	24.22
32.00	38.00	21.00	25.97	17.00	24.58
32.25	38.30	21.25	26.28	17.25	24.94
32.50	38.59	21.50	26.58	17.50	25.31
32.75	38.89	21.75	26.89	17.75	25.67
33.00	39.19	22.00	27.20	18.00	26.03
33.25	39.48	22.25	27.51	18.25	26.39
33.50	39.78	22.50	27.82	18.50	26.75
33.75	40.08	22.75	28.13	18.75	27.11
34.00	40.37	23.00	28.44	19.00	27.47
34.25	40.67	23.25	28.75	19.25	27.84
34.50	40.97	23.50	29.06	19.50	28.20
34.75	41.26	23.75	29.37	19.75	28.56
35.00	41.56	24.00	29.68	20.00	28.92
35.25	41.86	24.25	29.98	20.25	29.28
35.50	42.15	24.50	30.29	20.50	29.64
35.75	42.45	24.75	30.60	20.75	30.00
36.00	42.75	25.00	30.91	21.00	30.37
36.25	43.05	25.25	31.22	21.25	30.73
36.50	43.34	25.50	31.53	21.50	31.09
36.75	43.64	25.75	31.84	21.75	31.45
37.00	43.94	26.00	32.15	22.00	31.81
37.25	44.23	26.25	32.46	22.25	32.17
37.50	44.53	26.50	32.77	22.50	32.54
37.75	44.83	26.75	33.08	22.75	32.90
38.00	45.12	27.00	33.38	23.00	33.26
38.25	45.42	27.25	33.69	23.25	33.62
38.50	45.72	27.50	34.00	23.50	33.98
38.75	46.01	27.75	34.31	23.75	34.34
39.00	46.31	28.00	34.62	24.00	34.70
39.25	46.61	28.25	34.93	24.25	35.07
39.50	46.90	28.50	35.24	24.50	35.43
39.75	47.20	28.75	35.55	24.75	35.79
40.00	47.50	29.00	35.86	25.00	36.15
40.25	47.79	29.25	36.17		
40.50	48.09	29.50	36.48		
40.75	48.39	29.75	36.79		
41.00	48.69	30.00	37.09		
41.25	48.98	30.25	37.40		
41.50	49.28	30.50	37.71		
41.75	49.58	30.75	38.02		
42.00	49.87	31.00	38.33		
42.25	50.17	31.25	38.64		
42.50	50.47	31.50	38.95		
42.75	50.76	31.75	39.26		

Abdomen		Right thigh	
Inches	Constant A	Inches	Constant B
43.00	51.06	32.00	39.57
43.25	51.36	32.25	39.88
43.50	51.65	32.50	40.19
43.75	51.95	32.75	40.49
44.00	52.25	33.00	40.80
44.25	52.54	33.25	41.11
44.50	52.84	33.50	41.42
44.75	53.14	33.75	41.73
45.00	53.44	34.00	42.04

Appendix D
Oxygen and Energy Production

Breathing, heart beat, urine formation, and other life-sustaining functions are often taken for granted. Yet these vital processes require energy even when a person is at rest or asleep. The body forms and stores energy by means of a complicated series of chemical reactions called *glycolysis*—the breakdown of glucose, ultimately into carbon dioxide and water. This process requires oxygen. Glucose is readily available: It can be made from substances stored in the body. But oxygen must be continuously obtained from the environment in precisely the amount needed at precisely the time it is needed.

When you inhale, oxygen enters your lungs, passes through the thin membranes that line the tiny air sacs of the lungs, and enters the bloodstream. There it combines with hemoglobin in the red blood cells and is carried through the bloodstream to all the cells of the body. When the oxygen in the cells has been consumed during the process of glycolysis, the waste products of glucose breakdown are picked up by the blood and delivered to the lungs and the kidneys for elimination from the body. With every exhaled breath, then, carbon dioxide and water are returned to the air—along with any unused oxygen. It is therefore possible that cardiorespiratory endurance can be adversely affected by a lower concentration of oxygen in the inhaled air (as at high altitudes), by certain lung diseases that interfere with the transport of oxygen into the bloodstream, or by anemia (a decrease in the number of red blood cells).

Getting oxygen from the air into the bloodstream is the function of the entire respiratory system from the nose to the tiny air sacs of the lungs. Distribution of the oxygen to the cells of the body is the job of the cardiovascular system—the heart and the arteries (blood vessels). The heart is composed almost entirely of specialized muscle fibers. It contracts more or less rhythmically and steadily about 90,000 times each day. Each time the heart muscle contracts, blood is pumped out of the chambers of the heart into the arteries. During relaxation (between beats) oxygen-poor blood enters the right side of the heart from the veins of the body. From there it is pumped into the lungs to receive oxygen from the inhaled air. This blood, now rich in oxygen, returns to the left side of the heart, from which it is pumped into the arteries for delivery to all of the body's organs and tissues.

Just how much oxygen you need is directly related to your current level of activity. When you are resting or sleeping, your activity level is minimal. Because less energy is required, less oxygen is consumed. Your breathing rate is slow and shallow and, therefore, less air is inhaled. Your heart pumps more slowly, and less oxygenated blood is circulated through your system. During mild activity your oxygen consumption goes up because functions requiring oxygen increase. As long as sufficient oxygen is supplied to the cells, then aerobic metabolism—the complete conversion of glucose into carbon dioxide and water—can continue to take place. When the activity becomes more intense, and the supply of oxygen can no longer keep up with the demand, glycolysis continues up to a point. This incomplete breakdown of glucose, called anaerobic metabolism, results in the accumulation of lactic acid, which is normally produced but rapidly disposed of when there is adequate oxygen. The presence of increased amounts of lactic acid in muscle tissue may be a factor in fatigue and exhaustion.

When the activity level drops, everything gradually returns to normal. In order to repay the oxygen debt incurred during the period of anaerobic activity and to dispose of the accumulated waste products of glucose breakdown, the heart and lungs continue to work at elevated rates for several minutes after completion of activity. This is the recovery time. Eventually, aerobic metabolism is restored, the accumulated lactic acid is disposed of, and the sensation of fatigue is relieved.

Index

Index

Paperbounds from Consumer Reports Books

Physical Fitness for Practically Everybody. The Consumers Union Report on Exercise. 1983. $12

Love, Sex, and Aging. CU's study of sexual attitudes and activities of people age 50 and over. 1984. $14.75

What Did You Learn in School Today? Helping your child to do better. 1983. CU edition, $8.50

Guide to Used Cars. CU's reports, Ratings for '80–'82 cars; good and bad bets for '77–'81 cars. 1983. $10

Infants and Mothers. Advice to parents on baby's first year. Revised, 1983. CU edition, $11

The Food Additives Book. Safety ratings of additives in 6000 brand-name foods. CU edition, $10.50

Carpentry for Children. Do-it-yourself guide for kids who like to build things. 1982. CU edition, $10.50

Top Tips from Consumer Reports. How to do things better, faster, cheaper. 1982. $6.50

Putting Food By. The best ways to can, freeze, and preserve. Third edition, 1982. CU edition, $11.50

More Kitchen Wisdom. Another kitchen book from Frieda Arkin with more of her helpful hints and practical pointers. 1982. CU edition, $6.50

Consumer Reports Money-Saving Guide to Energy in the Home. CU's energy-saving strategies with product Ratings. Revised, 1982. $8

You and Your Aging Parent. Understanding the aging process; needs; resources available. Revised, 1982. CU edition, $9

Freedom from Headaches. For understanding and treating head, face, and neck pain. Revised, 1981. CU edition, $8

My Body, My Health. A self-help guide to gynecologic health for women of all ages. 1979, updated 1981. CU edition, $10.50

Child Health Encyclopedia. A comprehensive parents' guide. 1975. CU edition, 1978. $10.50

Kitchen Wisdom. Frieda Arkin's kitchen book to make it easier to cook, shop for food, and clean up. 1977. CU edition, $7

TO ORDER: Send payment, including $1.75 for your entire order for postage/handling (in Canada and elsewhere, $4), together with your name and address to Dept. BPP84, Consumer Reports Books, Box C-719, Brooklyn, N.Y. 11205. Please allow 4 to 6 weeks for shipment. Note: Consumers Union publications may not be used for any commercial purpose.